Rhema Yoga

Rhema Yoga: Stretchers One

ADAM MARKS

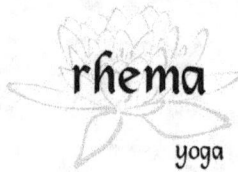

ISBN: 1536930253
ISBN-13: 978-1536930252

DEDICATION

This book is dedicated to my wife, Laura. Your encouragement, support and prayer has been both constant and vital in this long journey.

OTHER RHEMA YOGA BOOKS

Introduction Series

1. Rhema Yoga: Principles

Teacher Trainer Series

1. Rhema Yoga: Stretchers (1&2)
2. Rhema Yoga: Practices
3. Rhema Yoga: Jetpack
4. Rhema Yoga: Roots

BOOKS FROM THE RHEMA INSTITUTE

1. The Metron (Basics)
2. The Metron (Atmospheres)
3. Energy

CONTENTS

Stretcher: stretch·er. noun

3. A rod or bar joining and supporting chair legs.

Google definition of "Stretcher," retrieved in 2016.

MEET THE CLASS

The characters in this book are loosely modeled after 4 family members...

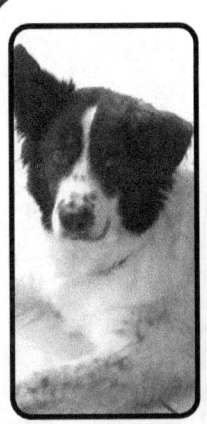 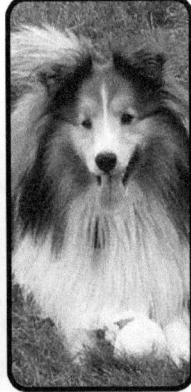 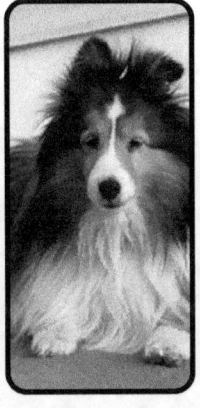 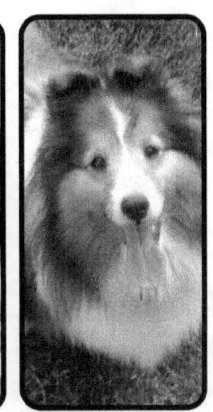

Sylvia	**Skye**	**Aurie**	**Bella**
-Rescued 10-yr. old Border Collie -Always hungry -Has been seen eating peas, carrots, noodles, lettuce, paper and butter -Lays by the front door for most of the day; unless anyone approaches the fridge	-Brillant Sheltie in the prime of his life (5 yrs. old) -Eager to please -Fits all standards of Sheltie looks, he is the "model Sheltie" in everyway -Would easily make it as a show dog -Has a loud, somewhat piercing bark that he loves to use	-Oldest, coolest Sheltie I know; 12 yrs. old -Very stubborn, slightly cocky -Not afraid to ask (aka: bark) for what he wants, for as long as needed -Loves to be around people, but expects service.	-Possibly the most nervous, anxiety-ridden dog I have ever met. She has a great heart and loves everyone -The term "licking machine" would easily apply to Bella the nervous licker -Barks at anything that moves, both in the real world and in her imagination.

ACKNOWLEDGMENTS

I would like to thank my wife, family and fellow Christian yogis. You have provided support, encouragement and even editing expertise throughout this entire process. I couldn't have done it without out all of your help!

CHAPTER 1

WHAT'S THE POINT?

You rush into class about 20 minutes late, hoping you won't be noticed. You're heart sinks when you look inside and find that not only are you noticed, but the entire class stops and looks at you. "Sorry... the traffic..." you squeak and hurriedly sit down. Adam, the guy who got you interested in all of this Rhema stuff with his book "Principles" just smiles, as usual.

"No worries! You get a free pass on the first class, but I'm going to give you an assignment for next week... don't worry, I'm not mad at you, I just don't want to do it myself. You gave me the perfect excuse!" He smiles again, and you nod unhappily as you sit down in a desk near the front. "Oh – one sec before you sit – you missed introductions, so would you mind standing up and telling people where you are from, what you are looking for from this class, annnnd... you favorite food?" You nod, jumping up to your feet again. You've been in enough of these classes to know the drill by now, and rattle through the list pretty quickly. The only thing that really is on your mind now is that extra assignment. Adam continues with what he was saying before you came in.

"So this class is called 'Stretchers' and it's a fundamental piece of training for anyone wanting to get started in their advanced study of Rhema Yoga. This is your foundation, your support for everything else." As he is speaking he begins handing out a short packet of papers, and you get yours from the girl sitting in front of you, holding pizza in her right hand and your now-greasy papers in her left. You thank her and look around the room for the first time.

It's everything you remember about old-school college classrooms. A white-ish tile floor, and a huge, somewhat battered white board. Pulsating, sterile fluorescent lights above wash out as much color as they can. The class is small. "Probably because Rhema is such a new thing" you decide, and has only four other students besides you. One is the girl in front of you, chomping down on her pizza and holding a Snickers nearby for a follow-up snack. Another is an older guy, about 60 from the looks of it, who is covered in tattoos, black leather clothing and chains. His leather-ish skin is crowned by a green Mohawk, of all things, that sits above two heavily pierced ears. He catches you staring, and you quickly look down towards your packet to begin reading. You'll have to take a look at the other two later, you decide. Adam seems to have given everyone some time to read, so you get to it.

~~~

Today there are so many different flavors of yoga in the marketplace, and thousands of books for each flavor. You might ask – "Is there really a need for another book about how to do yoga? What's the point?" That's where we are going to start off in this "Stretchers" lecture series.

What's the Point?

The point of Rhema is to develop a relationship with the God of Israel. This relationship is one that empowers students to live lives of joy and hope, confident in their identity as sons and daughters of a

> Our mission is to develop the son or daughter within you, and have a good time doing it!

royal family. Everything within this system of yoga is aimed at that relationship. As such, one of the sure signs of a Rhema Yoga yogi is a deep knowledge that we live from God's love, not for it. We do all things from relationship with God, not for it.

~~~

You put the first piece of paper down and notice another girl in the class who is sitting in the front row and on the far left. She seems to be nervous, afraid, and also a little annoyed. It's as if she has something on the stove that she needs to get to but can't until her question is addressed. Adam is at his old, yellow metal desk at the front of the classroom reading a book and doesn't notice her until she clears her throat.

"Um, teacher?" she asks. Adam smiles and raises his eyebrows.

"If I'm not flexible enough, can I still do this yoga thing?" The old dude next to you grunts with a bit of mockery, and another guy at the front of the classroom laughs a bit. Adam stands up and heads towards the middle of the room.

"A lot of people, and I was once one of them, have a belief that if they aren't already flexible, they really should not and probably can not do yoga. They go to a few classes and look at the people better than them, and think 'man, this is not for me.' It's a little like going to a gym and seeing a lot of fit people. You don't realize that they are fit because they go to the gym a lot, you just start comparing yourself and feel like you don't belong. I totally get that."

"First and foremost, an awesome benefit of yoga is increased flexibility and mobility. It's much like those people at the gym who don't seem to need the exercise. If you do it, you will get it! If you feel you aren't flexible, yoga would probably a perfect thing for you to do in order to become more flexible. Does that makes sense?" The girl nods, but then puts her hand up quickly.

"But, I mean, there's a lot more to yoga than standing on one leg, or doing the perfect handstand, or putting your feet behind your head." Adam nods in agreement.

"Absolutely! Well, especially in Rhema, which is different than a lot of other yoga systems like Bikram or Power Yoga that you've heard of in the past. Truth be told, a lot of people who are doing Rhema Yoga are more flexible than I am, and more experienced in teaching as well."

"What's that all about?" asks the old dude, forgetting to raise his hand. Adam sits down on the corner of his old, somewhat dented yellow desk.

"This is something I admire them for – they're amazing! I see their abilities and level of excellence and keep them in mind for my goals in my own practice. It makes me better. But amazing poses have very little to do with the other modules of Rhema, and they are all part of our yoga system. The girl looks confused, so Adam picks up a marker and writes on the white board:

"Are you Alive?"

"Don't worry about whether or not you're flexible enough to do Rhema Yoga. If you are alive, the answer is 'yes,' you have all the flexibility you need! This isn't a competition, it's an act of worship and a time of inner growth. It doesn't matter how old you are, how inflexible you are, if you have a disability, if you're not double-jointed, or if the shape of your bones is different than everyone else."

"Stick with a regular physical practice, and you'll see your body transform into something stronger and healthier, just like a magic trick, right before your eyes. Your mood will improve, your energy levels will increase, your confidence will soar, and I bet a whole lot more will happen too! Everyone is different, but there seems to be a lot of good for everyone who gets into a regular practice. Studying the 'Physical Body' module of Rhema Yoga in a consistent way will have a profound affect on the way your body feels and functions." The old guy raises his hand this time, asking his question while his stand is still going up.

"So what about all the pretzels then? It's not really yoga if you aren't able to do any of the poses." Adam stands up and starts going back to his chair.

"Feel free to look at the human pretzels of the yoga world as people to emulate to some degree, that's cool and I do it all the time; but keep in mind that you may never be as flexible or as 'bendy' as they are, and that's just fine. God doesn't care, and you probably shouldn't either. He created us all, body soul and spirit, in a unique and wonderful way, and this is all about celebrating that. This is not acrobatics. This is yoga. Rhema Yoga!" The old guy leans back into his chair.

"Uh... okay." He starts reading again. Adam bites his lower lip a bit.

"The word 'yoga' might mean something very different to you that it does to me, I get that. It has many different definitions in many different books, read in many different countries. For Rhema Yoga, it is defined to mean "Union, coming together, and uniting" with God. That's what you read about in 'Principles,' that book you had to go through before you could take this lecture series. I personally believe that this is also the most common terminology around the world, and that is one major reason I chose it instead of 'Rhema Stretching' or 'Rhema Postures' or something like that. It's true that it can be confusing for some people to use the word 'yoga,' but that just means we get to educate them later on." He smiles, and the old dude gives him a half smile before looking back to his paper packets. You were wondering if there was going to be a walk-out or a verbal spat, right there in the tranquility of the yoga lecture. No such luck. You go back to your reading as well.

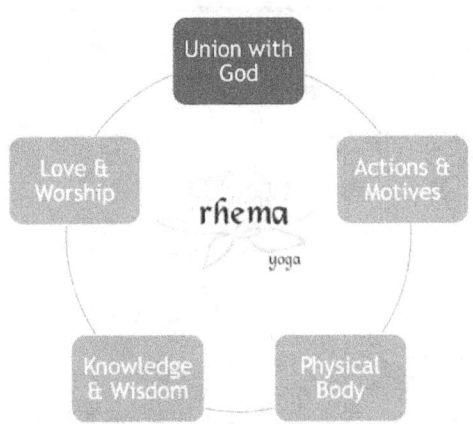

If you were just coming to Rhema Yoga looking to get into shape through postures, the nearby chart of modules might seem overwhelming. You may wonder "Where do I begin here?" or "What's the right way to do all of this?"

The answer, thankfully, is simple: anyway you want!

You could begin with the physical body module, but you could also start with worshipping and loving God, or searching for greater knowledge and wisdom with the Lord. The body of Christ is made up of many different people who have many different giftings, and each person has a module they will feel naturally drawn to. Where do you begin? It really depends on what you want to do, and it really doesn't matter what order you take. Everyone is different, and that is what makes us so powerful and wonderful as a body of believers.

I remember hearing a story in Elementary School about how we were all like the snowflakes that fell in December. Each snowflake was beautiful, mysterious and unique, just like us. We didn't have to be the same, even though we all felt peer pressure to fit in. Different "snowflakes" are designed with different destinies, and that's what the 5 Modules is all about. Rhema Yoga understands that we are all made perfectly and wonderfully by a loving God, and everyone should have a path to greater health.

> The more we learn who God is... the more we learn who we are...the more we learn to love life.

So each destiny will tend to draw someone more towards one or two modules much more than the others. You may enjoy the Knowledge and Wisdom module, while someone else loves the Physical Body module. But here is an interesting and wonderful catch: as one progresses into their module of choice, they will almost always find that their initial interest in one module will lead into another. I may start with the Physical Body module, but slowly migrate to the Knowledge and Wisdom module because of discoveries I have made about myself while performing different postures. This is because the modules overlap to some degree and are designed to reflect an aspect of both ourselves and our creator.

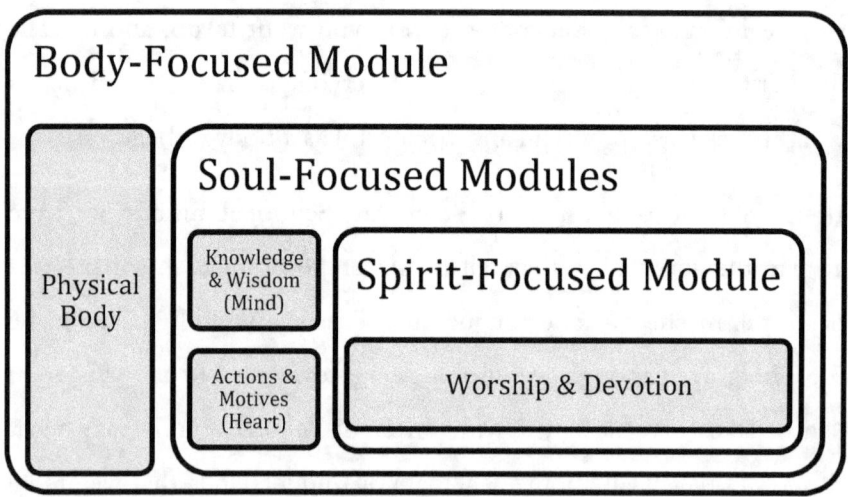

So feel free to smile, chose a module, and progress at whatever pace you prefer. There is no "you should start here" or "you should be

totally dedicated there." The only "should" I'll suggest to you is that you should have fun doing what you're doing, and you should only start somewhere if that module seems interesting to you.

I often suggest people develop a practice that touches each module to some degree, but again, this is only as a suggestion. The reason I recommend it is simple; most of us are currently only living one or two of the modules naturally, and often not completely. That can be limiting in our walk here on earth because each module is a way to know and connect with God. You've possibly had friendships where you only connected to someone in one area, but you've probably never had fulfilling and lasting ones like that.

This is much like speaking to a friend about sports and fitness, but nothing else. Perhaps your friend and you know all of the stats about the New York Yankees baseball team. You both know past, present and future stats. You know the stars, their stories, and everything else. You may chat for hours about the Yanks, and love every minute of it. But if that's all you ever talk about, you don't really know this person or have a deep relationship with them. How do they feel about politics? Art? Music? What are their values? If you only connect to this friend of yours through sports, then you only know this one facet of their personality. Everything the two of you do and say exposes only your opinon about sports, and particulary one team in sports. Many people know God this way. They pray to him or relate to him on one or two areas of interest, and then go hang out with other people for the rest. Hanging out with freidns and family is good, I just see an opportunity for deeper connection with God too.

Rhema Yoga has the 5 Modules because they allow an easy path for you to connect to God with your complete being. This allows us a way to know God intimately. Speaking with God and relating to him within the 5 modules leads us on to the path of becoming our full self, as we were designed to be. Nothing sets us up to achieve our destiny better than this!

So there are areas, or modules, of interest that we can use to connect to God with. What then? How do we do it? What methods can we use? In Rhema Yoga, the primary methods we use to connect to God are called the 4 Legs. These are postures, breathing, meditation and teachings.

> You can imagine the "4 Legs" of the chair sitting on the floor; the floor is made up of the "Modules."

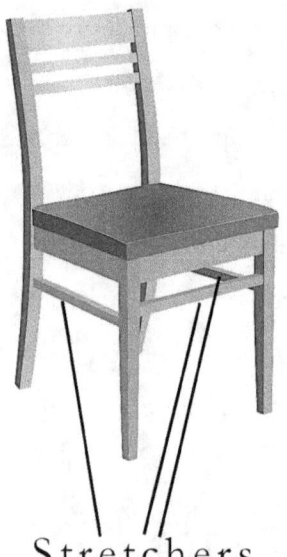

Stretchers

The legs are similar to the modules in that there is no particular one that you should do, or any specific order your should follow. As with the modules, everyone has their own preference, but people tend to do them all to some degree. This lecture series is not about the 4 Legs; they are addressed in detail in another class, called "Practices." This series is about the fundamentals of Rhema Yoga that fit in between the 4 Modules and the 4 Legs, called "Stretchers." As luck would have it, there are... you guessed it, 4 of them as well!

Why do I call them "stretchers," of all things? Well, part of the reason is because I like the double meaning of a chair stretcher and a yoga stretch. Another, much larger reason, is because the function of a chair stretcher is very much applicable for the "stretchers" we are about to talk about in Rhema Yoga.

A stretcher is the horizontal support element of a chair; it supports the legs of the chair, which support the seat. Indirectly then, stretchers support the entire seat of a chair as they directly support the chair legs. So it is with Rhema Yoga. The stretchers indirectly support your union with God as they directly support your posture, meditation, breathing and study practice. When we put all of the components of Rhema Yoga together, we come up with something like this:

The Rhema Yoga Structure

1. The Floor: The (4) Modules
2. The Stretchers: The 4 Stretchers
3. The Legs: The 4 Legs
4. The Seat: Union with God

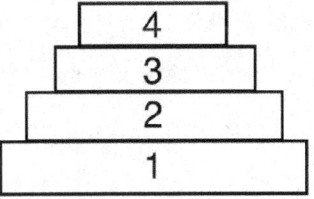

These are the four major structure titles of Rhema Yoga, which are all comprised of four elements, with the exception of the last component, Union with God. On a personal note, it was a fun coincidence to see the number 4 all over Rhema's structure. "4" seems to be heavily related to the concept of creation by many scholars. There are four great elements (earth, air, fire, and water)

four rivers of Eden (Genesis 2:10–14), four Angels (Revelation 7:1-4), and four Living Creatures (Ezekiel 1:5-10). It was on the fourth day that God completed the material universe. This is the day that God brought into existence our sun, the moon, and all the stars.

> *"Then God said, 'Let there be lights in the expanse of the heavens to separate the day from the night, and let them be for signs and for seasons and for days and years; and let them be for lights in the expanse of the heavens to give light on the earth"; and it was so. God made the two great lights, the greater light to govern the day, and the lesser light to govern the night; He made the stars also. God placed them in the expanse of the heavens to give light on the earth, and to govern the day and the night, and to separate the light from the darkness; and God saw that it was good. There was evening and there was morning, a fourth day.'" Genesis 1:14-19, (NASB).*

So it seems that the number for represents creation, and creative works. I like the idea of "creation" and the "Idea of 4s" in Rhema Yoga because we are recreating ourselves into sons and daughters. We are creating a bond and connection between us and God. We are creating a piece of heaven on earth with our practice.

The "Idea of 4's" in Rhema Yoga is easy to understand. We become new creations with the 4 Modules, 4 Stretchers and 4 Legs!

Here is a more detailed look at the Idea of 4s in Rhema Yoga.

The Floor: The (4) Modules

1. Knowledge & Wisdom
2. Physical Body
3. Worship & Devotion
4. Actions & Motives

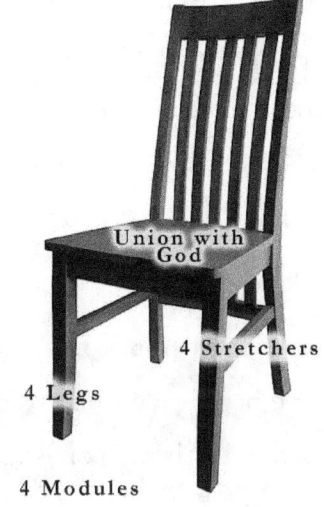

The Legs: The 4 Legs

1. Meditation
2. Breathing
3. Postures
4. Teachings

The Stretchers: The 4 Stretchers

1. Posture
2. Cleansing
3. Alignment
4. Locks

The Seat: Module 5; Union with God

~ ~ ~

You put down the papers from your reading as Adam starts drawing out a soccer field. "If you have a hard time understanding how the modules, legs and stretchers all work together, think of the following soccer analogy. It helps me a lot. Pretend you are a soccer player. As a soccer player, you know you want to win a game (Union with God). To do that, you need to score goals, which means you need to shoot the ball, pass the ball, dribble the ball and head the ball (the 4 legs). In order to do these things well, you'll need to practice a lot, work out a lot, eat well and study game plans (the 4 stretchers). Of course, all of these things are useless unless you know where the soccer field boundaries are, where the goal posts are, where the goalie box is and what the rules of soccer are (the 4 modules). Everything has its place, everything builds off of each other." You try to write it all down, but get lost in all the soccer verbage.

"One last thing before you go, and it's a big one, so write it down and remember it. We won't really take time to dig into it until later in this series, but it will come up from time to time in many of our classes. First, there is yoga sonship, and secondly is yoga orphanship."

"Yoga sonship is a term to describe a balance of stability, ease and tension in the body and soul when you are doing your yoga practice. A yoga pose in sonship has stability and ease for the yogi performing it, and not excess tension. Sonship allows someone to enjoy their practice because it's fun, and they feel their body becoming healthier in the process – there is no place for striving and straining in any part of your being. Yoga orphanship, by contrast, is all about excess effort, focus on others and not yourself, comparison and more. It results in tension and disease, and it comes with a much greater possibility of injury. Does this all make sense?" You don't understand what he's talking about, but you managed to get it all written down, so that's a start. From the corner of your eye, you notice that several people have begun leaving class for the day.

"Hey teach" the man next to you is standing and still staring at his paper. "That chair on the last page only has three stretchers… did you know?" He's smiling, and the rest of the room lets out a chuckle as they start packing up. Apparently they noticed as well, but didn't say anything. Adam laughs, and picks up his paperwork to take a closer look.

"Right you are, Aurie, thanks for the heads up." You get up to leave with the rest, but then remember that you have a homework assignment due next week because you were late.

"Maybe he'll let me off with a warning" you think to yourself, grabbing your bag and heading up to the front of the room.

CHAPTER 2

THE ENEMY: FORWARD HEAD, PART 1

You jump in through the classroom door, about five minutes late, hoping you aren't spotted. Adam smiles and asks you to come over to his desk. You look around, happy to see that not everyone has gotten into their seats yet. You may be late, but at least you didn't stop class this time!

"Do you have the assignment I gave you?" he asks hopefully. You smile and nod, handing him several large, colorful drawings you made over the week. "Wow! These are awesome! A lot more color and pizazz than I would have used – thanks!" You smile again and skip a bit as you head over to your seat, the same place you were at last week. You decide that the pictures make up for being late last week and lean back in your chair, content with yourself and eager for today's lesson.

"Last week we discussed a lot of the theory and structure of Rhema. I wanted to give you an idea of how it was built, and where you are now in your course of study. All of that is useful in helping you understand *why* the topics we are about to study are valuable in your yoga practice. For this week, we're going to move on with a chat about one of Rhema Yoga's biggest enemies; Forward Head Syndrome." Adam starts handing out more papers at this point, and you grumble a little bit when you get yours. If you wanted to just read about yoga, you would have bought a book or something.

You take a look at the handout, and start reading.

~~~

Forward Head Syndrome

What a title! "Forward Head Syndrome." It almost sounds like a scary disease out of Star Trek or something. Unfortunately it is all too real, and has been with us for centuries. It is especially prevalent in the west, where we slump over steering wheels to drive our cars, hunch over phones to text our friends, squint at computers to write books (like this one!) and more. Almost everywhere you look, you'll see people with forward head syndrome (FHS). In fact, you might have it yourself – right now – as you're reading this! Before we get more into the details of what FHS is, lets talk quickly about the spine.

The human spine has a handful of natural curves, three of which make up an "S" shape when left in a healthy, neutral state. For the sake of our study, we are going to be studying these three curves more closely. They are critical in

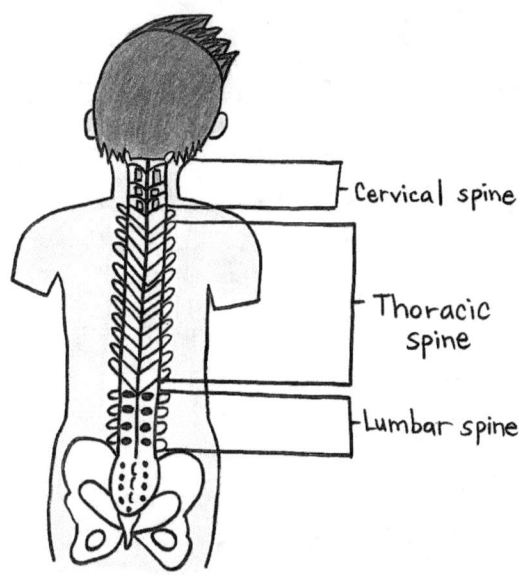

understanding FHS and what it is, as well as how to resolve it. The more you learn about these three curves and FHS, the more your posture practice will begin to provide greater benefits to your physical and emotional health.

~~~

You flip the handout over and are happy to see that it's blank on the other side. "Okay" you think to yourself, "I guess a little reading isn't so bad to start off with." Adam waits until everyone seems done with their papers before he continues.

"Does everyone understand the handout? Does anyone have any questions?" No one raises their hand, so Adam continues. "Great! In that case, lets go ahead and talk about the three major areas of the spine. Bella, do you have your homework done for today?" You look over to the nervous girl sitting up at the front-left side of the classroom, and watch her as she anxiously gets out of her seat and begins to walk up to the front. When she reaches the head of the classroom, she turns and begins to read mechanically from a paper that she is clutching in both hands with an iron death-grip.

"The top part of the spine is called the cervical spine, or cervical curve. This is your upper spine area, and it makes up the top of the 'S' shape that our backbone looks like. The cervical curve includes what many of us know as the 'neck' area." She looks up from her paper to the class as if each person in the group has a rifle pointed at her head. With a gulp, she continues reading. "The cervical spine naturally curves inward. That curve inward happens in a concave fashion." Her fearful monotone is starting to put you to sleep, so you begin hoping she's almost done. "The Cervical section of the spine has a lot of mobility. It can twist quite far."

"Good job Bella! That is a pretty good intro to the Cervical spine." As he speaks, Adam is going through the small stack of colored illustrations you created for your homework, and you realize in horror what is about to happen. Sure enough, he pauses in his search through the pile of drawings, squints his eyes a bit, and then decides to put one of your pictures up onto the white board. You want to hiss at him and throw your pen, but decide to stay quiet. So far, no one has really laughed at your creation, so you decide to play it cool until they do.

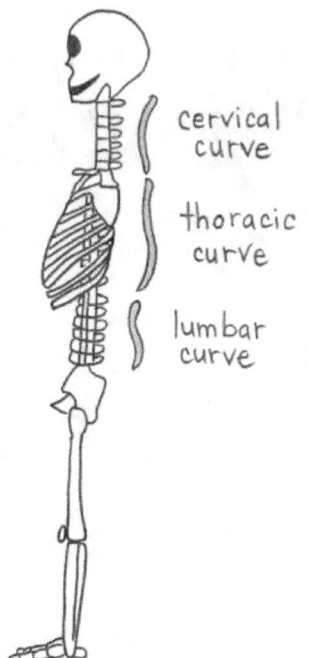

cervical
curve

thoracic
curve

lumbar
curve

"If you look at the picture up here, you can see the cervical curve of the spine sitting up at the top, where our neck is." He points to the picture. "Okay, good. Bella, can you continue?" Bella's face looks horrified at the suggestion, but she swallows hard, and turns back to her paper. Soon that robotic, monotone voice starts again, but you notice a few less quivers of terror in her tone as she begins.

"Next is what is called the thoracic curve. This is the middle of the back or spine…" she nervously and rigidly motions towards your picture "…as you can see, it is attached to the rib cage." Bella looks in Adam's direction and he smiles and nods, so she continues with a bit more confidence. "This section of the spine would normally be very mobile, but the rib cage hinders some spinal rotation." Adam clears his throat and interrupts.

"The thoracic spine is a very important region in Rhema Yoga. A large portion of our poses are aimed at either rotating or bending the thoracic in a way that counters forward head." He turns back to Bella. "Great job so far, what else do you have?" Bella's eyes widen and she drops her head to her paper again quickly.

"The thoracic spine is convex in its curvature." She looks up again. Adam turns towards the picture.

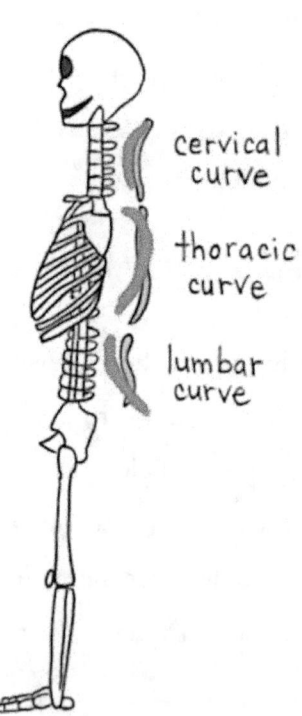

cervical curve

thoracic curve

lumbar curve

"Oh… right… well, you can't really see it here in the picture…" you start clutching your pen, ready to pounce at the first chuckle. "The spine makes that 'S' shape we mentioned earlier, and that is because the cervical curve is concave in nature and the thoracic curve is convex in nature." Adam grabs a large, red marker and starts drawing on your work of art. "Something a little more like this… yea… here is what the spine actually looks like." You want to rip the picture down and tear it up into a million pieces, but decide for now that the information is too valuable and jot it down in your notebook. Bella continues her reading.

"The lumbar curve, or the lumber spine, is our lower back." Adam interrupts again.

"Right! The lumbar! This is a key part of our back in Rhema Yoga as well, but for a different reason. Whereas Rhema focuses on bending and twisting the thoracic, many other forms of yoga focus on bending and twisting the lumbar. That is why the lumbar spine is the part of our backs that many of us 'crunch' in our backbends and overextend in twists. So for Rhema, remember this important bit – we are mostly about getting *out of* the lumbar and getting *in to* the thoracic when it comes to twists and bends. That is one thing that makes us different from a lot of other yoga systems. The lumbar, like the cervical, is concave in its curve, but unlike the cervical it is the least mobile of the three in terms of bending and twisting. Therefore, we focus on *gently* twisting and bending there only!"

"A good way to teach twists is from the ground up, because it allows us to focus on not crunching or over-twisting the lumbar. One thing that you'll want to remember in regards to twists in the lumbar is that the average rotation for a person's spine is less than 90 degrees." He stops, looks around the room, and decides to add a bit more. "That's 90 degrees… This will most definitely be on the test so write it down!" You pause for a second. No one told you there was going to be a test! "Go ahead Bella." Adam says. She looks at him like a cornered animal, and says nothing. "Is that all you have left about the lumbar?" Adam asks. She nods yes, and Adam lets her sit down.

"Good! That was a really good introduction to the spine and it's three major sections. Thanks to our classmates, we were able to learn about it all through both presentation and illustrations. As we said, there are other sections of the spine besides these three, but for the scope of this lecture, we are really only interested in the thoracic, cervical and lumbar. The Rhema Yoga book 'Yog(a)natomy' goes into much greater detail about the spine, should you want to know more, but if you only know about these three, you'll be just fine." You write down the name of the book for reference just in case, but don't feel your heart race with excitement at the prospect of buying and studying an anatomy book. You haven't yet lifted your gaze from your notebook when another handout is on your desk. The room is quiet as people begin to read it, and you reluctantly begin to do the same.

~~~

When someone has FHS, the symptoms are obvious. Their chin juts out over their chest, and their chest is both sunken in and hollowed back. Their ears are not aligned over the shoulders as they should be, but are instead ahead of them. This is because the chin is jutting out, over the desk. What of the shoulders? They are slumped forward as well. Notice the picture of a person slumped over their computer.

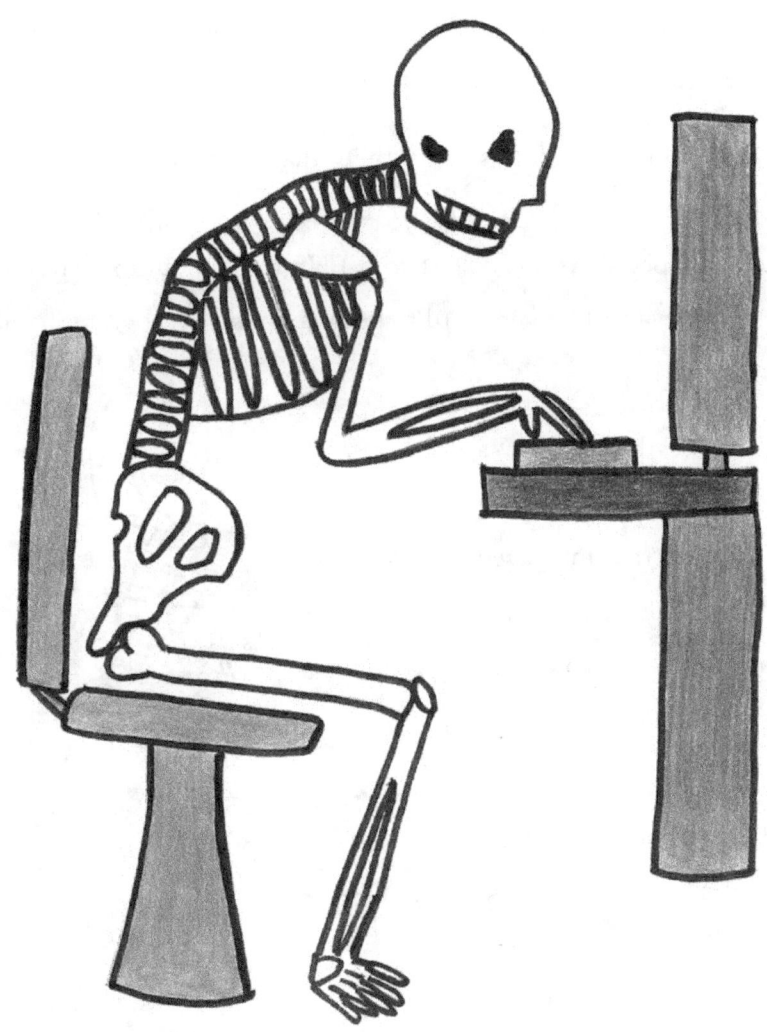

This sort of position puts a lot of strain on the neck and shoulders that was never meant to be there. Suddenly, your neck and shoulder muscles are doing all the work! Whereas the head is meant to balance at the top of the spine, it is suddenly hanging out and over, like a gigantic piece of fruit on a small branch. There, your shoulders and neck are the only thing really holding the head, a ball of ~10lbs. up in the air. As you might imagine, this poor posture is one of the most common causes of neck, head and shoulder pain in the western world today.

It's prevalent too. FHS is not a thing that only video gamers and authors deal with. I challenge you to go out into public and see how many people you can spot with FHS throughout the day. My guess is that it will be very hard to keep count all day, because you'll see so many!

In the nearby picture a person is sitting in a chair at a lecture; that may even be how you are sitting right now! If you look closely, you can see very clearly what were talking about. Notice that when the thoracic spine bends *more* into its natural curve the cervical and lumbar spine *go away* from their natural curve. This is how 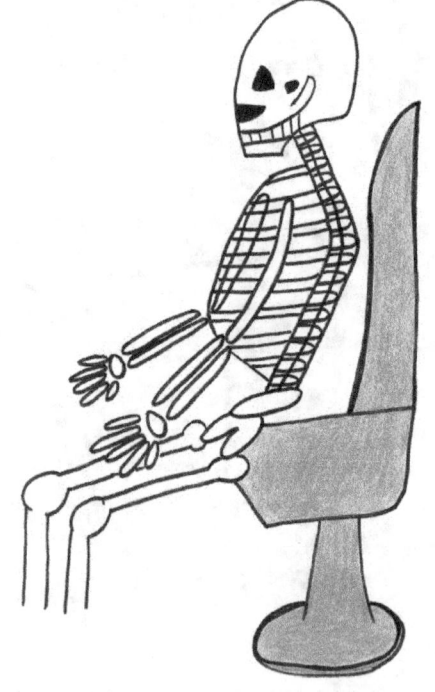 the spine works, it's general mechanics. None of it is a major issue however until it becomes habitual, forward head syndrome. FHS is why so many people in the U.S. today have lower back problems when they get older, as well as those aches and pains in their upper back that I mentioned earlier. It's all a common effect of poor posture, and it's one of the big things that Rhema Yoga addresses.

> Some negative *physical* affects of FHS include long term muscle strain, disc herniation and pinched nerves. Decreased respiratory strength and chronic neck pain have a strong correlation with FHS.

When we say that our goal in Rhema Yoga is to be both physically and spiritually aligned to God, posture patterns are at least half of what we are talking about. Surprised? Don't be! FHS has negative affects on all levels of our being, and I believe you'll see what I mean over time. Suddenly, the old school teachers who would scold their students for bad posture don't seem so bad, do they?

~~~

You lift your head to see what's next, and find the rest of the class still reading. Adam is walking over towards the girl in front of you, and whispering to her while pointing towards the whiteboard. She nods a few times, and he starts back to his desk. Apparently there is yet another homework assignment that is going to be presented to everyone. After a few minutes more, the rest of people in the room lift their head, and he continues.

"We've hit the end of our time here in class today. Next time we meet, we'll wrap up our discussion with a presentation from Sylvia."

You pack up your things and head home for the day, interested in the idea of FHS and determined to fight it off.

CHAPTER 3

THE ENEMY: FORWARD HEAD, PART 2

"How many of you looked around to see if anyone was sitting in forward head this week?" Adam asks, raising his hand up at the same time. Skye raises his hand, but no one else does, and you quietly give him the label of "teachers pet."

"Cool! Did you count a lot of people Skye? I'm going to guess that if you did this, you stopped counting pretty quickly because so many people in the U.S. do it!" Skye laughs and agrees heartily, and you phase out the jovial conversation that follows as the two enjoy talking about how prevalent forward head is in America. After a few minutes, the focus shifts away from Skye and over to Sylvia, who puts down a box of cracker jacks when she notices Adam gesturing in her direction.

"Lets finish off our talk on FHS by diving in to some of its negative affects, starting with the physical. Sylvia is going to help us there." Sylvia walks to the front of the room and prepares to present something to the class. Unlike Bella, the girl from last week, she seems almost bored with the idea of speaking in front of the group. You get your pen ready as she begins.

"One negative affect of FHS that we should all be aware of is poor permanent posture. When an incorrect posture is practiced every day, throughout the day, for many years, the spine will begin to adapt. It will take on the shape of that posture more permanently.

It is good for everyone to remember that the body is very shapeable, and changeable. So if we have FHS all the time, the spine will adapt to FHS in a permanent way." She pauses, and you're not sure if it's for effect or because of confusion. "When we are in forward head posture, the spine experiences pressure in different parts of the vertebrae than those it was meant to. When a more permanent FHS posture is adopted because we are habitually in forward head, that pressure in different areas of the spine has an impact that gets worse and worse. Over time, FHS will slowly influence the spinal curves to change their positions permanently… or… or at least semi-permanently. That's when serious injury occurs." Adam steps forward a bit to add on to what was just said.

"Sylvia is right. One key thing to remember is that permanent changes can be made in the spine because of habitual pressure being applied to areas that are not made to handle so much pressure. Are you with me? As those areas of the spine adapt, there is a cost. Often, this is the sort of thing that leads to a herniated disk, but it could be even worse. Keep in mind that your spine is specifically designed to help absorb shock and keep you balanced. If your spinal position changes in a permanent or semi-permanent way, your natural ability absorb shock and stay balanced becomes compromised. More dramatic injury suddenly becomes likely, because your entire spine is now out of alignment. Not exactly a warm and fuzzy thought, huh?" Bella laughs nervously, and Sylvia continues reading.

"Another consequence of FHS is poor breathing. Forward head

negatively effects the breath; as the thoracic spine moves more into its natural curve, the shoulders collapse forward. The more the thoracic spine curves into its natural curve, the more the shoulders slump. This slumping of the shoulders makes the front of your body close up and hollow out. That closing and hollowing out action makes it hard to take full deep breaths." She looks up quickly to see if her words are having an impact, then looks back down to her paper.

"So, when you go to the doctor's office, you may hear them say 'Sit up straight and take a deep breath.' One reason they do this is related to what I am talking about. It isn't just because they need to put their stethoscope on your chest and hear your heartbeat. They also need to be sure that your lungs and diaphragm, among other parts of your torso, are free to move as designed. That is one way they can tell that you are able to breath deeply." You suddenly remember Broadway plays and operas you went to a few years ago, realizing they always had great posture when they sang. In order to sustain a note or have a powerful voice, they must need to train themselves to stand up straight. You quickly jot the thought down in your notebook, next to a doodle of an opera singer. Sylvia continues her report.

"The last physical problem I found related to FHS was nerve pain..." at this point, Adam cuts in quickly.

"If you've ever heard the phrase 'pain in the neck' then it might take on a new meaning here! A lot of us think that FHS causes pain in the neck because we are overworking our muscles. After all, it was just last week that you read about how the head is a heavy ball you should be balancing on top of your spine. That's true, but it's not just about overworked neck muscles. When in we hang in slouch mode, vertebrae can more easily be pulled out of alignment. Over time this will cause what will at first be gradual, and then more painful nerve impingement." Aurie sits up in his chair after almost falling asleep in the last few minutes.

"Impinge-what? What is that?" he asks, almost seeming upset.

"Nerve impingement. In this case, it means having a pinched or irritated nerve in the neck. I'm saying that this nerve can get pinched or irritated because the spine slowly starts to fall out of alignment, and then hits the nerves there. As soon as that happens, you'll know it right away because it will cause pain, numbness, and weakness that will actually start to radiate into the chest or arm areas. That will wake you up to the world of posture patterns right away! Many times people hear of shoulder impingement, but it can absolutely happen near your neck too, because of FHS." Adam looks away from Aurie and back to Sylvia, who is returning to her chair in front of you. "Is that all Sylvia?" She nods yes, and as the class claps, she sits down. Adam begins to talk again.

"I have two more possible affects of FHS that I'd like to suggest for you all. They are digestion and constipation!"

"Ewww!!!" Bella throws her pencil down causing Aurie to laugh.

"Right – sounds gross to some people." Adam continues. "It really is just a natural human function, but yea, it can be nasty I guess, so let's get constipation out of the way first."

"Believe it or not, even your 'bathroom breaks' can be negatively impacted by a slouching forward head posture. Who would have guessed it?" Adam pauses and looks around the room, which is quiet except for your muffled chuckles. Your laughing more at Bella's response to the topic than the topic itself. Adam continues.

"When you sit in a crouched position your intestines are essentially folded up…" Aurie interrupts Adam here, arm raising as he speaks.

"What else is new? Haven't you seen a human diagram of intestines before? It's like ramen noodles in there!"

"Uhh… well, yes… let's say that they fold up even more than normally. They get really folded up in a bad way, and that restricts your bowel movements. When I was in China they often used squatty potties, where you just sort of squat over a hole in the ground. One of the major reasons for this sort of potty is for reasons related to what we're talking about here. It was gross, don't get me wrong… especially when someone had terrible aim and no desire to clean up after themselves; but squatting down is somewhat practical because it actually opens your intestines and increases the likelihood of bowel movements."

"It's not practical for me!" Aurie interrupts. "I don't think I could squat like that and do my business even if I wanted to! And definitely not if someone can't hit the target! Who cleans that up!?" Adam makes a strange face.

"Well that's a good question. I know someone must have, but they didn't seem to come around often to do it… it could be pretty nasty. I never really got the hang of it, and judging from the poor aim that some people had, they never did either." Bella has reached her breaking point here, and raises her hand.

"Can you guys please-please move on?"

"Right, sorry. Anyway, it may seem unlikely, but the truth is that if you have FHS for an extended period of time, you may find yourself developing issues with maintaining a healthy bowel movement."

"Which leads us right into our next topic, digestion. When you consider the how closely the stomach and intestines work together, it only makes sense that digestion could be affected by FHS as well. Poor posture has been found in many cases to dramatically slow down both digestion and bowel movements. Making small, healthy changes in your posture is a good thing for your digestive system and worth the time and effort to do."

"So lets go ahead and write out a quick list of what we've said so far." He turns to the whiteboard, grabs his big marker, and lists out the following:

Posture, Breathing, Nerve/Muscle Pain in the Neck, Digestion, Constipation

"Good!" he says, putting the marker down and spinning on his heel towards the class. "Now that we've said all of this, it's time to move on. You may want to make a note of the list above though, because it highlights the importance of healthy posture for your physical body."

"With your body experiencing so many aches, pains and discomforts, you can imagine how FHS may also adversely affect your soul as well. Our bodies and souls are interdependent, they are connected in ways we cannot really even begin to understand. FHS will affect your mood, your perception of yourself, your perspective of the world and of other people around you. Not only that, it also affects the way that others perceive you!"

"Extensive studies have been done that show how the leaders in a group almost always have a healthy posture, while most followers take on some form of FHS, even if they didn't have it in the past. Job interviews and business deals are very often dictated by non-verbal communication related to posture as well."

"Amy Cuddy, a Social Psychologist at Harvard Business School, has done a lot of really cool research in this area, and two of Rhema's postures are taken from her work. She talks a lot about how body language can change people's perceptions and even body chemistry. That means both our confidence and our cortisol levels. This all bleeds into every facet of our lives, as you can imagine. Everything from self-image, moods, emotions, relationships, and more are affected."

Skye raises his hand at this point. For the first time, you take a good look at him. He is about 25 years old, sports long blonde hair, and seems to have muscles on top of his muscles. You can more easily see him surfing than teaching yoga, and decide that he may be doing both.

"What is it, Skye?" Adam asks.

"What moves did you make up in Rhema Yoga based on her research?"

"The Rhema pose called 'superhero,' which is in many of our sequences, was one of them. 'Victory pose' is the other. You'll see

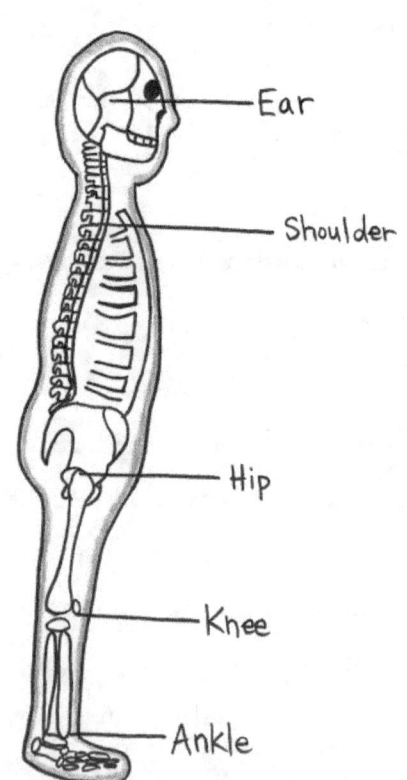

both of them when you take some more of our classes, or if you decide to study the 'Practices' workshop in a few months." Adam begins rifling through your pictures again, and you see him take the other one you made, tape it to the whiteboard, and continue teaching.

"The cure for FHS is Optimal Standing Posture (OSP), which is what this drawing is supposed to be illustrating. The body is standing strong

and aligned. That's 'OSP.' Are you loving these acronyms yet?"

"When you consider OSP, think about Mountain Pose, because it's the perfect illustration of what OSP looks like. Your hips are over your ankles, your shoulders are over your hips, your heart (and chest) are positioned forward, your ears are over shoulders and your chin is slightly tucked. So OSP is the cure for the national ailment that most people in the U.S. have, called FHS."

"When we are not in optimal standing posture we are usually in FHS, and that's where the problems begin. There are other postures that are also unhealthy, but again, the vast majority of people in this country suffer from FHS. That's why Rhema Yoga considers it to be one of our biggest enemies. In the end, it doesn't really matter if you have FHS or another unhealthy pattern, either way our muscles are suddenly finding themselves with demands to do things they weren't designed to do. In FHS they begin working harder just to hold up the head and keep the spine stabilized and protected, all at the same time. This is a lot to ask your body! Hold up a 10 pound weight you weren't designed to hold up, and then stabilize and protect the spine as well? Tall order!" Adam stops to take a drink of water.

"Sorry, I know I'm talking a lot now but there is a lot to cover before we finish today." He points to your drawing again before continuing. "All the extra work that your body has to do causes muscle tightness, soreness and fatigue. So as you may imagine, it's not a stretch to assume that FHS can affect mood, energy levels and stress. If your body is not happy, your soul is going to feel it!

Some negative *soul* affects of FHS include feelings of depression and decreased energy. People who slouch had a 10% decrease in testosterone and a 15% increase in cortisol (a stress hormone) in several recent health tests. Why is that important? It basically translates to into low self-confidence and high stress.

All of these feelings can be reversed by living in a more upright position." He looks over at your drawing again, pulling out a large black marker and grabbing the same red marker that he's been using so far.

"This is an awesome drawing, but there are a few mistakes here. Can anyone see it?" You raise your hand quickly.

"The spinal curves are off, like they were in the first drawing from our class last week" you say quickly, just to make sure the class sees that you know your mistake.

"Good! That's the first mistake." Adam makes corrections with his red marker. "Anyone see the other?" Your face flushes. Another one? Skye raises his hand.

"The person is standing on a slant. He's not straight up… no knees over ankles and shoulder over hips and all that." Adam nods.

"That's it! Good job Skye!" Skye smiles, and Adam starts making the changes.

"Good! So the curves are a little different, and that big black line I made should go from the ears, through the shoulders, hips, knees and ankles if they are all aligned and stacked on top of each other. Does that make sense?" Everyone nods. "Still, these pictures are really well done. Great job everyone!"

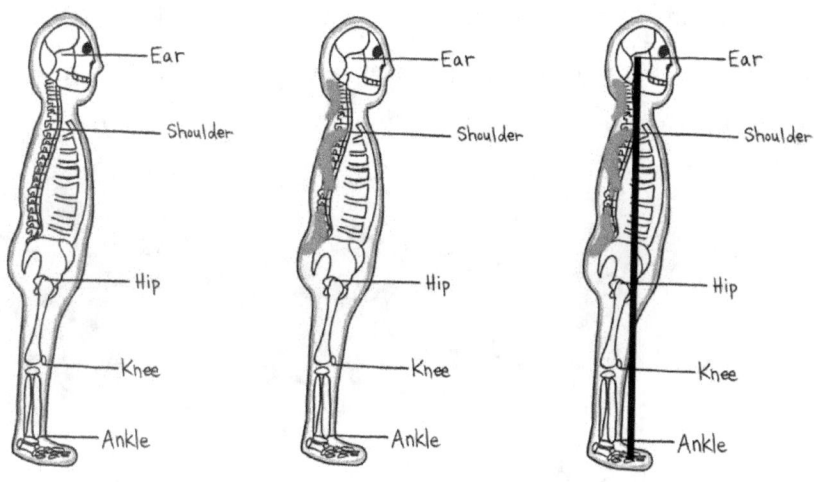

"We have less than five minutes left in our class, so let me finish up on OSP now. Maintaining OSP may not be the first thing that comes to mind when we think about Christian Yoga. It probably isn't even close to something you'd think about when you consider issues such as career, the digestive system or self image. The truth is that there are massive long term benefits in becoming more physically aligned, and these benefits affect every area of your life. As such, you'll notice every pose in Rhema Yoga consider proper alignment and optimal standing posture. It doesn't matter if we're talking about Crescent Lunge, Warrior 2 or Bridge." Bella starts packing up, and Adam glances to the clock. "Oh gosh! Okay… well, one set of very important tools that helps us find and maintain

OSP is the muscle locks, which we will discuss next week. I know we ran a little late today, but I appreciate you all sticking around and letting me finish up. Have a good week guys and girls!"

You close your notebook and start packing up. Overall, it wasn't a bad class, but you don't remember as much as you would have liked to. You decide to go home and review your notes a few times as you get ready to go.

CHAPTER 4
THE MUSCLE LOCKS, PART 1

You enter the classroom 20 minutes early this time, proud of your planning prowess and ability to avoid rush hour traffic. You're the first one, and decide to review some of the FHS/OSP material from last class. As you cover the information, you suddenly realize that you haven't thought about FHS all week, and have probably been sitting in the unhealthy posture the whole time. Quickly you sit up into OSP, but after a few minutes tire and slump a little. So begins your struggle to sit upright for the rest of the class.

Eventually the rest of the students file in, Aurie being the last one, and a few minutes late. He sits next to you again and gives you a "hey" when you glance over to him.

"Hi" you say, in your best "I'm-cool-too-but-I-don't-care-about-it-as-much-as-you-do-so-I'm-not-going-to-put-as-much-effort-into-my-'hi'-that-you-did" voice. Adam begins writing on the board:

The Muscle Locks

"Hi guys an girls! Welcome back to another lesson. Ready to get started?"

"Let's do it!" shouts Skye, sitting straight up in his OSP at the front of the class. Adam smiles, and the lesson begins.

"Okay good – we're going to spend our next two weeks on the muscle locks. Altogether, there are seven muscle locks that you'll

39

want to memorize for the test in Rhema Yoga. I don't just want you to commit them to memory though, I want you to understand them fully and learn to incorporate them into your practice, if not your daily life. How many of you had a hard time sitting or standing in OSP this last week?" You quickly look at the four other students. Sylvia has one hand up and another on a cheeseburger, Skye's hand is down, Bella is nervously lifting her hand ½ of the way up and mumbling something anxiously, and Aurie is looking at the white board like he wants to punch it. You didn't really have a hard time sitting in OSP because you totally forgot to try, but if you had remembered, you definitely would have struggled at it. You decide to join Bella and Sylvia, and slowly raise your hand.

"Good! I mean, I understand where you are coming from if you had a hard time doing this. Today I'm here to help with that, and muscle locks are how. There are seven in total that we will consider for Rhema Yoga, and they are foot lock, root lock, ab lock, full ab lock, throat lock, hand lock and soul lock."

"When learning these, I always recommend that you begin with throat lock, and the three most important locks to me are soul lock, throat lock and ab lock. Root lock comes in closely at fourth place. Traditionally muscle locks they are thought of as energy locks. When we engage the muscles associated with the lock, the force created helps stabilize our bodies in our pose. For example, when we use foot lock in mountain pose, the force created rebounds up our inner thighs and reaches our core to ensure a strong, well-aligned mountain pose. When we engage the locks in everyday life, they help correct our posture, especially if we are dealing with habitual forward head. So as you can imagine, muscle locks are key actions that should be applied in every active yoga pose."

"When we are in our downward-facing dog, the force created from hand lock actually does rebound up our arms to stabilize them. It sounds funny or silly, but it really helps. Not only does it stabilize our arms, but hand lock also brings the weight of our bodies out of our wrists and up to our shoulders. That makes down-dog a lot healthier! Does all of this make sense so far?" Adam asks. The room is silent, although you have a feeling it's because people are a little lost and don't want to admit it. You decide to speak up.

"I don't understand how flexing some muscles can help us stand stronger or straighter... that doesn't make sense to me" you half-heartedly admit. Adam smiles.

"I felt the same way when I first heard about locks. Don't worry, it will probably become clear as we go into detail about each one." You nod your head, and Adam starts taping up a picture of a massive foot on the whiteboard. You look over to Skye's notes to see him diligently sketching it out, and decide to do the same. Aurie yawns and leans back into his chiar as Sylvia begins opening a bag of saltine crackers. Adam pivots suddenly on his back heel to face the class again.

"Okay, so we'll start from the bottom up, with foot lock first." He smiles, apparently happy with what may have been a joke he just cracked. You play with your pen nervously as you decide whether

41

or not you should fake-laugh. Sylvia stuffs a saltine cracker into her mouth and Skye looks down very intensely at his notes. Adam moves to the picture of the feet he just taped up and points to the many labels.

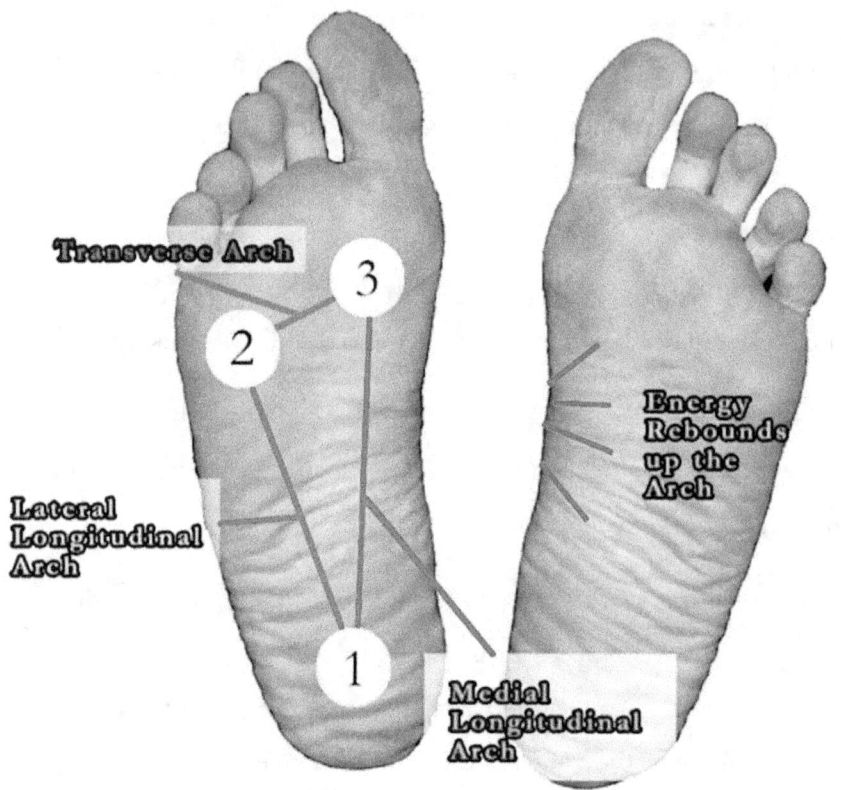

"First off, don't worry about remembering all of these titles... it would be helpful in our teaching if you knew them, but it's hardly required. It took me awhile to remember them myself, and if I wasn't teaching, I don't think I would!" He pauses to put down his markers before continuing.

"These three points on the sole, numbered 1-3 on the diagram, represent the parts of your foot that you want to consider the most when performing foot lock. Here is where your pressing down to the earth. Basically, you are rooting down on '1' and the space between '2' and '3' for your lock. When you do it correctly, muscle energy will rebound up the inner arch, or 'Medial Longitudinal Arch,' all the way up to your pelvis area. That goes a long way in adding stability to your poses, especially standing poses like tree, mountain, dancer and superhero."

"Your inner arch, or 'medial arch' is that part that is higher than the rest of your foot. It's full of elasticity because it is so much higher up than the other arches and because it's made up of so many small joints. This arch is full of soft, elastic tissues that work to act like springs when we stand, walk, jump or more. In fact, when you walk or run, the impact is spread out and recycled for a bigger bounce because of this arch. That energy 'bounce' can be used to stabilize us in our postures, and that's the bounce that we're going for with our lock. The transverse arch, at the front of your foot, is important for rooting down in foot lock, but the medial arch is important because it's where the energy rebounds upward."

"To repeat, when we contract the muscles in foot lock, we find that stability that we need because this action provides extra force to bring stability in the body. Does that make sense? It will definitely be on the test! Foot lock is vital to all of our standing poses, as you can imagine, so it's important to both know how to do it and why. You want to try to remember to do it throughout your practice."

"So how do we do it then?" Asks Aurie, hand raised.

"Glad you asked. It's easy enough, as are most of them. To start off, root through the center of the heel and…"

"Sorry… do what through your heel, now?" Asks Aurie again, arm still raised and brows furrowed. You're not sure if you like this guy, you decide, but the question is a good one. What in the world does "root" mean, anyway?

"Root" replies Adam quickly. It means engage the muscles at that location and draw energy from the action. Often times, that location is pressed down to the floor, but this isn't necessary. For foot lock, think of a tree with roots deep and wide. Your toes are wide, your sole is planted… you're rooted to the ground, just like a tree. Your foot is touching the floor in it's key locations, and the muscles there are contracting and engaged. You should get a better idea of what I'm talking about as we continue. Sorry, I just don't want to go too far off on a rabbit trail here – I tend to lose my train of thought, and we need to cover all of this stuff today." Aurie nods, and the class continues.

"So you're going to root down through the center of the heel in the back of your foot. In the front, you're going to root down on the meaty flesh that's behind the middle toes. Between the big toe and the pinky toe mound of the foot, all that space roots down, or is pressed down by you… got me so far?" He looks at the class, and specifically Aurie, before moving on. "Okay, so in Mountain pose, the center point of the heel roots down into the ground with the front of the foot. As you push down you want to create the rebound, or lift of force, that travels up through the medial arch, inner thighs and into the pelvic floor. This force, or energy, should help stabilize the body and begin to engage the core muscles as well."

"Foot Lock is more important than you may think, so don't underestimate how much it can add to your practice like I did when I was first learning yoga. When foot lock is used correctly, it will allow many alignment actions to automatically happen, making poses easier and better. It will also make OSP much easier to maintain." Adam looks at Sylvia, who is now loudly crunching saltines, seemingly forgetting where she is at the moment as her pen lies half buried in a small mound of crumbs on the floor.

"Okay class, write these bullets down. Just in case you forget them or need a quick reference about foot lock a few months from now when you're making your class plan." He turns back to the whiteboard, and quickly scratches out the following in blue. Sylvia crunches down on a cracker before beginning a frantic search for her pen.

Doing Foot Lock in Mountain Pose

- Let your breath soften.
- Keep your toes spread wide on the mat.
- Do not grip the mat with your toes.
- Root down between the center of the heel and behind the middle toes

- Engage your inner thighs
- Knees should stabilize, check to be sure (we'll talk about how to stabilize knees later on)
- If you don't notice a difference and improvement in your balance when you start foot lock, you can improve something in your lock
- Engage root lock lightly, not with all your strength, as force rebounds up (We will discuss how soon!)

"Keep in mind that foot lock should be accessible to you at all times, whether your on the mat or in a subway train. It actually doesn't even matter if you're standing in tree pose with your feet on the mat or laying down in corpse pose with your feet in space. This is mostly about engaging your muscles, not about the earth being below your feet. When used correctly, foot lock will create the strong rebound of energy that helps your poses, and you'll actually feel it come up your inner thighs to your pelvic floor muscles. When the energy hits your pelvic floor, muscles there will contract lightly. That leads us to the next lock now, which is called root lock."

"Sorry" Bella interrupts. "Are we talking about the core? You're saying the pelvic floor. I don't quite follow."

"We don't have much time to get into this, but the pelvic floor is part of the core, and that is the part that we are discussing now. We'll get into more details later, so don't worry about it too much at the moment." Adam turns back to the board and continues the lesson.

"I'm not going to draw where root lock is on the body, because it's in a bit of a sensitive space. It's a vital lock for many postures, meditations and more though, so pay attention. Root lock engages the core muscles, activating and strengthening the deep core each time it is engaged. Because of that, root lock supports skillful, healthy body movements. One important thing to remember in Rhema Yoga is our belief that all healthy body movement initiates at the core. It doesn't matter if you are in class or real life. All skill-*full*, healthy movement, regardless of the pose, initiates from the core. If you engage root lock during your yoga poses, all of your postures will get an extra sort of lift that will make them seem easier and lighter to do. Even jumping with root lock feels totally different! If you guys ever remember when your outside of class this week, give it a try!" Adam looks down at a paper he has on the desk in front of him and begins reading. Apparently he's a bit lost in his notes.

"Root lock is all about guiding us to move more from our center, or our core, than from other parts of our body. This is important because any full body movement really should initiate from the core." He looks up to the class again. "Eh… sorry, we just said that. I sort of lost my place in my notes. Anyway, it's a good reminder! Healthy, skill-full movement starts at the core! Okay, lets see now… ah! When you start contracting the muscles involved in root lock, you become more and more aware of how the deep core of your body works. This continues through muscle sensations and noticed differences in your yoga poses. Such increased awareness will help you move more efficiently and fluidly both inside and outside of your practice. It will always work in your favor for better postures, more energy, and even injury prevention." Adam looks over the class now.

"Does all that make sense? Sorry there are a lot of things I just can't memorize, but I still want to say them just right. Do you all understand what I'm saying?" Sylvia raises her hand.

"I know you don't want to draw it, but where is this lock? How do we know how to engage it?" Adam smiles.

"Right, right, okay. The short answer is that root lock is like a web of muscles. This web is between your sitting bones and your pubic bone. When you slightly contract this web and lift it upwards, you are engaging root lock."

"Sitting bones?" Bella asks, putting her pencil down.

"Yea, that's not the technical term for them, but it's easier to remember."

"What's the technical term?" Skye asks, leaning forward a bit with his pen posed to write. Adam shuffles some papers on the desk.

"Uhhh... let me see... um... here it is! Ishial Tuberosity bones. Phew! Try saying that three times quickly! I prefer sitting bones. So the sitting bones and the pubic bone make a sort of triangle at the bottom, or 'root' of your pelvis. This is where your 'root lock' is located, the bottom of the pelvis." Sylvia puts down a granola bar she has just opened.

"Sorry, sitting bones? But where are they?"

"Ah... oh forget it, I have a few pictures here..." Adam begins another mad shuffling of his papers, which are beginning to slowly grow into a living, breathing, moving blob on his desk. "Ehh… let me find it now… Ah! Got it." He says, pulling a large diagram from the pulsing mass of papers. "Okay, so that's a good question Sylvia, and I remember thinking the same thing when I was learning about the locks as well. Here we go!" He does another one of those

sudden pivots on his heel and twirls around, taping the diagram up to the whiteboard in the process.

"These…" he begins, turning slowly around and pointing to the two lowest bones in the pelvis, "are the sitting bones. As you can probably tell, they are called sitting bones because you can feel them very clearly

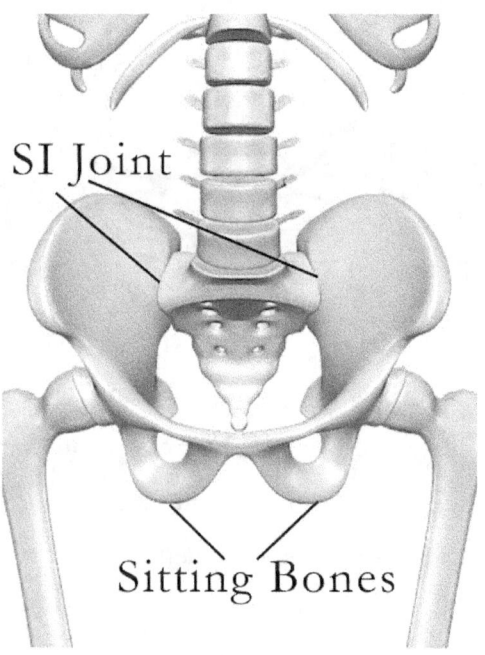

when you are sitting down on any surface, although harder surfaces are better." Skye raises his hand quickly, and Adam calls on him.

"I see the 'sitting bones' on your picture, but I don't understand what an 'SI Joint' is? Is that important for us to know?" Adam glances back at the picture and nods.

"Yep! You'll want to know at least a little bit about the SI Joint, but we won't talk about so much right now. Also, I don't have a picture of that besides what's up here already…" He picks up a black marker and sketches out a hip section on the white board. "Here you

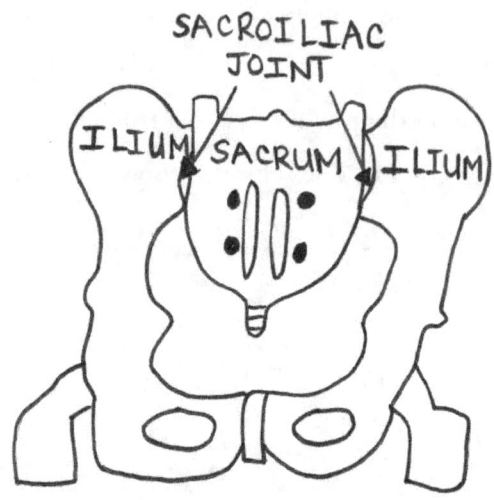

can see the sitting bones at the bottom, right?" He points to the two boney points at the bottom of the drawing and everyone nods. "The SI Joint is an actual joint that moves only a tiny bit, and it's between the sacrum and the illium in your pelvis. That's where the name comes from, actually. It's the sacroiliac joint, connected by strong ligaments. The sacrum is what supports your spine, and it's right below the lumbar curve. The sacrum is supported in turn by an ilium on each side. So the SI joint and the rest of that area is something important to us in Rhema Yoga, but it falls outside of the scope of these classes. For now, just go back to finding your sitting bones. Take a minute to try it out if you're not sure what I'm talking about. You have to sit straight up to feel your sitting bones the best, but either way you should feel them pretty quickly." He waits a bit as the class all starts squirming in their chairs, trying to find their sitting bones.

"The space in between the pubic bone and those two boney protrusions that I call the sitting bones is the pelvic floor. To engage the web of muscles in that space is to engage root lock. Got it

Sylvia?" She nods her head yes, and Adam continues.

"Okay cool. So just to make sure this is crystal clear, once you find your sitting bones, think about how those three bones form a triangle. Got it?" The class is silent, but Bella and Skye nod along with you, so Adam continues.

"Great. Now, I know I'm repeating myself over and over again, but I really want to be sure you know what I'm talking about here. Imagine that triangle we just mentioned, the one that is formed by the sitting bones and the pubic bone. Once you get it, we're going to go ahead and engage root lock for the first time. Ready? As soon as you feel good to try it, gently lift the muscles in this triangle."

"You should feel a lift in your core, throughout your torso. This is the sort of energetic lift that you'll be wanting to have when you're doing Rhema Yoga. It makes a big difference. I would suggest using it when you're doing life too — whether you're driving in your car, sitting at your desk, eating lunch at a café, or whatever. Just remember that whenever you are holding root lock for extended periods of time, you really only want to hold it gently at about 15% to 30% effort, no more. If you do it more, you won't be able to maintain it, and you might become rigid. This is just a light engagement of the muscles, as are most of the locks."

"For the women students who you are teaching root lock to, it might help to mention to them that this light lifting does include the vaginal walls. Guys, if you're not sure what I'm talking about, ask your wife or girlfriend or… whatever. It's important that you know what I mean and remember to teach it, because root lock is one that all of your students will benefit from."

"For you ladies, if you're familiar with Kegel exercises, root lock is basically that, but with a lot less effort. Go easy on me here, this is all abstract information for me. I haven't had any kids yet, so I have no experience in this area! In fact, I didn't even know what Kegel exercises were until I did some research. In case any of you don't know what I'm talking about, Kegel exercises were developed a while ago in the U.S. to help pregnant women prepare for and recover from childbirth, among other things. They strengthen the pelvic floor muscles and the action is quite similar to root lock. What you really need to know is that root lock is comparable to Kegel exercises, but different in that root lock requires only about 30% of the effort you would need for Kegel. Is that clear? So it's not about 'how much can I squeeze that web of muscles and pull them up?' It's just 15% to 30% of the effort. You engage the web and feel a gentle lift. As we mentioned before, when you do foot lock the energy that rebounds up your inner thighs will engage root lock for you, or at least make it easier to do root lock." Adam takes a deep breath before moving on.

"Gosh, we're running a bit out of class time here so I need to hurry. Why do we always run out of time?" Bella raises her hand nervously here, and Adam reluctantly calls on her.

"Sorry, I have to go soon. Class is already over and I need to go on errands." Adam nods.

"Well, I'll finish up the muscle locks next week. For now, remember what we talked about, and try to come to class early next week, I'd like to cover the rest of them so we can move on to alignment issues. We're a little behind in your course schedule as of now."

You gather up your notes and leave with the rest of the group, thinking of sitting bones, pelvic floors and Kegel exercises as you head on out towards your car.

CHAPTER 5

THE MUSCLE LOCKS, PART 2

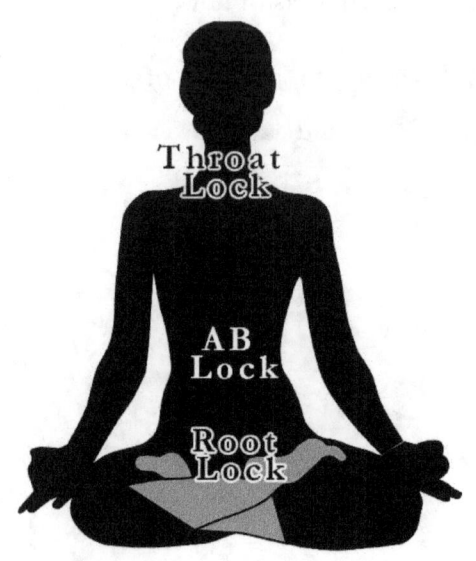

Things begin quickly the next week, and Adam walks over to the whiteboard to tape up the nearby picture exactly when class starts.

"So last week we discussed root lock, which takes place at the pelvic floor. This week we're going to start at the abdominal area with two locks called 'ab lock' and 'full ab lock.' You can call them abdominal lock and full abdominal lock if you'd like, but ab lock works just fine too, and it's much easier to say in conversation. Either way, we'll know what you mean."

"The point of ab lock is to activate the deep core, similar to the way root lock does. However, ab lock not only activates the deep core, it also supports and aligns the rib cage. When you engage ab lock, you are activating the lower abdomen muscles, and this is what brings support to the ribs. Here, you are drawing the rib cage in through the ab lock action. There are many yoga poses, such as down-dog, where we have a tendency to jut our rib cage out. Ab lock goes a long way in correcting that. Doing this lock is easy enough, and it brings noticeable benefits to your posture right away, so it's definitely something you'll want to incorporate in your practice."

"To do it, you want to scoop the tailbone lightly while at the same time drawing the belly button softly in toward the spine and up toward the ribcage. When you do this, you'll feel sort of a... like a deep contraction in your lower belly. This contraction in your low belly results in low back support. The support is strong and sudden, but not rigid. So your back will be stable, but it will still be flexible."

"When ab lock is performed correctly, you'll know it because you will feel a physical response through the body that allows for a whole laundry list of alignment actions to happen. You won't have to focus on them or make them happen either, they will simply fall into place. There's no need to memorize this list, I don't know it all myself. But it's good to write down for reference." He moves to the whiteboard and starts sketching out a list.

Automatic Ab-Lock Alignment Actions

1. The natural curve of the lumbar spine will appear
2. A widening will take place across your back body
3. The bottom front ribs will move in toward the spine.
4. Your core will stabilize through ab muscle engagement (This aids with balance and injury protection)

You scribble the list down quickly, unsure of what you're writing but determined to review it when you get home tonight. For now, it's all about copying things down.

"As we said before, the key to a good ab lock is to draw the belly button in towards the spine and up towards the rib cage. Similar to root lock and foot lock, this is also not a really strong, tight, or rigid contraction that you're making here. You not trying to tighten up the whole abdominal area, that would almost surely lead to excess tension and rigidity. So ab lock is not a full-blown, muscle clenching sort of action. It's a lighter, deeper contraction, just like the others. When you have all of the locks engaged, you are really just very lightly contracting key muscles in key locations. It is because the contractions are light and not at full strength that the locks are all possible to have engaged at once."

"For ab lock, you draw the belly button in and up and you just feel the deeper contraction in the abdomen take place. If it makes your whole waist feel rigid or tight, you're doing something wrong, and it probably means that you're using too much energy. Nothing about ab lock should make your whole waist feel rigid or tight. There will be times when applying the lock is going to require more effort, but even then you will not be engaging ab lock at your full strength." Adam stops and steps towards the class. "Can anyone think of a time when you might use ab lock with a bit more effort?" You look around at the others, hoping that if you look towards them, so will the teacher. It seems to work. "Skye? You have anything?" He shakes his head no, and Bella picks up a stress ball from her desk.

"Okay, no worries, I don't expect you guys to know, I was just curious" he smiles. The one situation that you'll want to use ab lock with a bit more effort is when you are in poses that have you working against gravity to apply the lock. This happens much more often than you might imagine. Postures like plank or downward facing dog all have gravity pushing your ab muscles down. With that being the case, it's going to be a little bit more effort to pull the belly button in towards the spine and then up towards the rib cage. You'll need to adjust accordingly to be sure that you do it, but not overdo it. Everyone is different in this area, and you'll find that many of the postures require a different amount of effort for different people. It's not too complicated though, and the most important thing is that you remember to try it when you do your poses. It will help to practice, and over time you'll really benefit from it." He moves back to his desk and begins shuffling papers before looking up again.

"We're going to move on now without time for questions. I want to get these locks done today and I only covered one so far! Next up, full ab lock."

"Full ab lock is actually a custom term that my yoga teacher made. I've adopted it into the Rhema Yoga system because it's perfect to describe what we're doing here. It's used to describe the original version of ab lock that was used for many centuries, and that most systems would call 'ab lock.' Rhema Yoga has taken another, different action to call 'ab lock,' which I just described to you, and changed the name of this traditional locking method to 'full ab lock.' I hope that's clear. So, the ab lock we have now is a much newer version that people found to be helpful in their practice. However, full ab lock shouldn't be forgotten."

"To do full ab lock, you want to breath in about ½ of your lung capacity, and then in a sudden, forceful exhale, breath all of the air out of your lungs. When I do this powerful exhale, I usually bend forward a bit and cave my chest in, almost like I'm doing a very exaggerated forward head. As soon as the last of the air leaves my lungs on my strong exhale, I close my mouth and do not breath in through either my nose or mouth. Then, I sit upright in OSP, and let a natural vacuum take place that sort of 'pushes' everything in my core upward."

"You don't want to hold your breath too long, but make sure you hold it at least for a moment. You want a rush of blood to move throughout your body when you release the natural vacuum you created with your breath so that the fresh blood washes all throughout your core, torso and organs. This is a unique lock because it is used for your cleansing practice, not your postures, meditations or other activities. So don't be too surprised to see that the methods you use to perform it are almost exactly opposite to those you use to perform the other locks. Whereas I've been constantly saying you should only use about 15% effort on the other locks, here you want to use maximum effort. Another thing that's different is that you're not going to hold this throughout your posture practice. Really, you're going to hold this lock for only a short time during your cleansing practice."

"We mentioned that a lot of people discover that ab lock takes a bit more effort to do in poses like downward facing dog. This is not the case with full ab lock. Full ab lock can be easier in down-dog because gravity is already working to naturally push organs within your core up to your chest. That being the case, it takes less effort to use the breath and perform the required actions."

"Phew! We are flying today compared to last week! How's everyone holding up? Are you with me?" Skye, Sylvia and Aurie nod, but Bella seems lost.

"I don't understand anything you just said about full ab lock" she says.

"That's okay, it can be a bit confusing, because it's so different. For now, just try your best to create that vacuum through a large exhale and by holding your breath. You'll get it if you stick with Rhema for any amount of time, and because it's a cleansing lock, you really don't need to know much about it as of now. We'll discuss cleansing practices in the second half of this series, and then full ab lock will be back on the teaching plan. For now, you can always reach out to me or the other people here. We have a lot more locks to cover, so we really do just have to keep going now. The next one is throat lock, and it's an important one to know!"

"Throat lock primarily involves your chin and your throat, but it works to improve your entire posture by bringing your head back and the heart forward. This lock is a key ingredient in fighting one of our biggest enemies, FHS. Luckily, it's easy to do."

"First you want to drop your chin slightly and then draw the base of your skull back far enough to keep your ears over your shoulders, so that they are aligned. When you do it correctly, you'll feel a physical response through the body that allows the heart to come forward softly and almost naturally, while at the same time your shoulders move back."

"As you'll recall, here in the U.S. we have that huge posture problem of slouching the shoulders and moving the head forward. Remember, that head of yours is a 10 to 13 pound ball of weight that was made to balance on the top of your spine. Reading books, watching TV and texting have us in FHS, with our shoulders rounded frontward, our heart caved in and our head hanging forward as well. Balancing your head in alignment, at the top of your spine is the ideal. This is OSP. This is what throat lock allows you to achieve."

"When we use throat lock, our head is no longer being held in space by a lot of our neck and upper back muscles, it's just balancing on the top of our spine, where it should be. The lock is really nothing more than a slight constriction that happens in the throat to move the chin back and down. Easy-peasy."

"Before we move on because of time, I really want to stress the importance of this lock. In Rhema Yoga classes you'll hear the cue 'move your ears back over the shoulders' for a lot of the postures. That's because taking the ears back over the shoulders as you pull the heart forward is another way to engage throat lock. It's very similar to the action of pulling the chin back and down. Saying it different ways helps more people understand what you are trying to do." Adam looks over at Bella quickly. "And what are we trying to do Bella?" She jumps a bit in surprise, dropping her stress ball in the process.

"Oh... well, throat lock helps put us back into OSP, which good. So we are trying to get students to use throat lock to fix FHS and do all of their postures in OSP."

"Right!" Adam says. "That's perfect! OSP is a healthy way to live both on the mat and off, and throat lock goes a long way in getting us there. I think throat lock and ab lock work really well in finding and maintaining good posture all day."

"Okay – two more to go! We've got just enough time left... ready to do this? Hand lock is next!" Adam closes a green notebook and opens a blue one, and a shower of papers fall out onto the desk. "Gosh... I really need to get things organized here. What a mess!"

"It's just creative genius!" Skye offers. Aurie scoffs.

"I'll go with that, Skye." Adam smiles. "Okay, hand lock. Here we go!"

"Hand lock is an action that is vital in protecting your wrists from harm. Many people who don't use it find their wrists hurting after a month or two of taking yoga classes, because basic poses like downward facing dog can really hurt the wrist joint. Using hand lock correctly will support and strengthen your wrists, and you'll also find your poses to be more aligned and easier to do because of it. Okay, so hand lock keeps you from pressing the wrists into the ground, hurting the joint. Ready for another benefit then? When you don't press your wrists and the heel of your palm into the ground, you avoid compressing the carpel tunnel." Adam looks around, but the room is silent, almost as if he had suddenly blurted something out in Chinese. "Eh… so, when we compress the carpel tunnel, we press on the nerves that run through that carpel tunnel, and that causes a lot of pain and stiffness in the wrist and hands. A lot of you have probably had this sort of condition before if you've used the computer with incorrect posture; as you know, carpel tunnel syndrome causes a lot of wrist pain. Has anyone ever *not had* carpel tunnel before?" Sylvia raises her hand, but everyone else keeps their hands down. "Yep, most of you have had it, including me. It's no fun."

"So hand lock supports the wrist and reduces compression. It also strengthens the wrist, which is going to be a huge benefit if you're doing a yoga practice with poses that require a lot of weight bearing in your hands. Besides down-dog, which we just mentioned, other poses would be plank, side plank and low plank; three poses that us westerners love to do. There also is all the small-dogs and toe-dogs that Rhema likes adding in. If you start to learn handstands and other poses like crow and firefly, you're really taking it to the next level. Those poses increase the amount of weight that you're bearing in the hands quite a bit. That being the case, hand lock suddenly goes from 'nice to know' to 'absolutely vital.' With me so far?" No one moves. Adam smiles, seemingly relieved, although you're guessing it's more because they didn't ask any more questions than anything else.

"So enough introduction, let's get on with how to do it. No one ever really imagines that something like hand lock would be needed, but man, we just showed how it is really vital to your practice! When you do it right, your wrists and even the rest of your body will feel a lot better in the long run!" Adam raises his palms now so that they are facing the class. "To start, you're going to always want to remember to root down through the heel of the palm. Bella – what does it mean to 'root down' in our locks again?" Bella is quick to answer.

"It means that this is the part of your body where your muscles are the most engaged. It also can mean that most of your weight is placed here." Adam nods.

"That sounds pretty good. In the case of hand lock, you are engaging the muscles in the heel of the palm as you root down through that area, but you are not putting all of your weight into the heel. So you root down there *as well as* the front pads of the hand and the finger pads, and there is where much of your weight is. Again, I know I said root down through the heel of the palm, but don't be confused. It's really important to make sure you don't get confused and think it's okay to collapse your weight into the heel of the palm. This is a common mistake that brings a lot of wrist pain. You *do not* put all of your weight in the heel of the palm. You *are* rooting down through the heel of the palm, which means you are engaging muscles in that area of the hand, but you *are not* resting on that area. In fact, hand lock is just the opposite of resting on the heels of your palms. Most of your attention is directed at pressing into the base knuckle of the index finger and the inner heel of the hand." He pauses for a second, just to make sure everyone is thinking about what he just said. You underline it in your notebook.

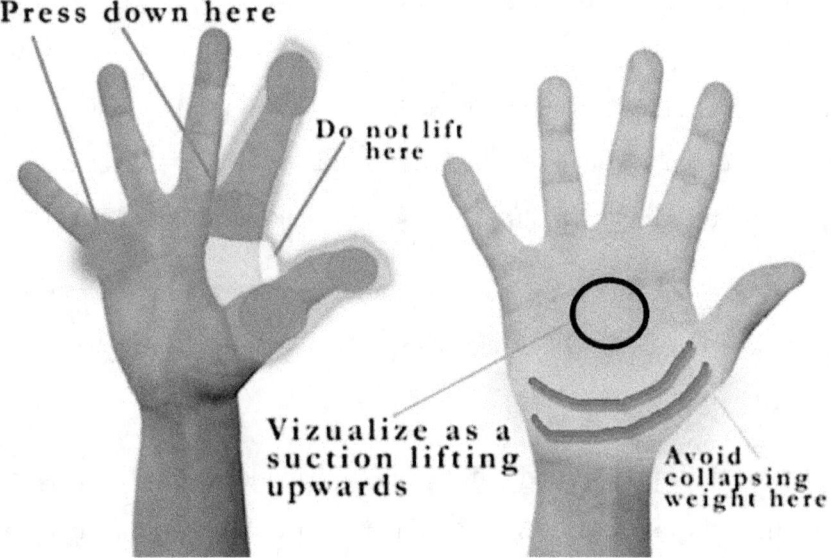

Press down here

Do not lift here

Vizualize as a suction lifting upwards

Avoid collapsing weight here

"Meanwhile, the middle of your palm is almost like a little suction cup. This suction cup action happens as a result of your muscles being engaged, causing muscular energy to rebound up. So, far from just resting on the heel of your palm and developing wrist issues, you're using your muscles to root through the heel of the palm, the front pads of the hands, and the finger pads."

"This makes hand lock an energizing lock, and when you do it correctly, you'll actually feel a sort of 'rebound' of force travel up through the arms. That force really helps you automatically make actions and key alignments for your postures." Sylvia puts down a twinkie she had just bitten into and raises her hand.

"What sort of key actions and alignments?"

"Good question, Sylvia! Hand lock brings about an internal rotation of your forearms and an external rotation of your upper arms. That's one reason it is essential to do a good hand lock when you perform small-dog or down-dog. In these poses, remember that hand lock leads to a decompression of the carpel tunnel, that trouble zone we discussed earlier, but it also simultaneously lifts and hollows the armpits. Hand lock begins at the hand but it translates to the rest of the body and helps build a healthy down-dog. There are many other poses that benefit from a good hand lock too, besides the two 'dog' poses we just mentioned. Examples could be those I mentioned earlier... handstand, plank, low plank and side plank."

"It's key to remember that hand lock is something you're going to want to apply any time you hands are in contact with the ground. It's similar to foot lock in that it supplies that stability, alignment and energy that we just mentioned, so you will benefit from using it regularly. You root your hands down, and then you press through the front of the palms and inner heel. Simple as that. Just be sure that you always press through the space between the thumb and the first finger – that is the part of hand lock that I personally focus on the most in all my poses. As you root down there into the floor and rebound up through the inner and outer arm, you'll feel the power bring stability and alignment to your pose. If you're in a handstand or something like that, you'll really notice a big difference. In these poses, your body continues to reach in the direction that the arms are reaching, so it's best for your alignment and stability if you continue that rebound all the way upward."

"I have no idea what you're talking about right now" Aurie admits, not at all happy about it. "I feel like your just repeating yourself over and over, but I don't know what you're saying…. How do I have any control about where the force or energy or whatever rebounds or doesn't rebound?" Adam nods.

"I try to repeat key lessons bits and reword them as many times as possible, to increase the likelihood that you'll remember them, so bear with me if it gets annoying. As for the whole idea of energy rebounding this way and that, I totally understand what you mean there. I'll admit that when you're doing this, a lot of it is in your mind as much as it is in your body; but that doesn't mean it is less valid or doesn't work! If you don't feel like you understand what I mean, or how you could ever do what I'm talking about, just imagine it happening, and try a little bit to make it happen. Over time, you'll notice it happening more and more." Aurie seems unimpressed.

"Let me try again." Adam says, turning to the board and drawing a stick figure doing yoga. "Here's an example - in downward dog, if I'm rooting down through the front of the palms, using my inner heel of the palm and then the space between the thumb and the forefinger, I'm doing a good hand lock, right?" Aurie nods. "From there I rebound up, through the inner and outer arms. I'm actively pushing into the earth, and I keep taking that lift up, through the whole torso. Even if that lift comes up only in my imagination, that's okay. Over time, my body will start to find ways to make such a lift happen, even if through subtle muscle movements. Energy goes further up through the side body, and I keep lifting as long as I can, through the side of my body and up through to the hip joints. Hand lock creates a stabilizing, aligning force of energy as I push away from the ground with my hands. That energy is traveling all the way from my hands to my hips to create a powerful, stable, straight back." It all started with hand lock. Aurie raises his hand for another question, but Bella speaks first.

"Time's up teacher, I have to go!" Adam glances quickly up to the clock.

"Oh shoot! Okay Bella, give me 5 minutes or less, please?" Bella, already halfway out of her chair, reluctantly nods and sits back down. You wonder if she actually enjoys the classes and learning about yoga or not. You suppose a lot of people sign up, not knowing exactly why or what they are doing, and regret it later. Adam interrupts your thoughts with a flurry of data that comes your way.

"Soul lock is the next and final lock we'll discuss for the Rhema Yoga muscle locks. It's a huge one too, because if you remember to do it, it will prove to be one of your absolute best tools for doing poses in a state of yoga sonship, not orphanship."

"Soul lock is all about the tongue, believe it or not. When you use this muscle correctly, it supports a balance of effort and ease in the body that helps you enjoy your practice, not become injured through it. By doing soul lock throughout your postures, you'll find that you have a built-in sonship meter, providing feedback of when you are using excess effort. It's like a 'son-o-meter.'"

"To do this lock, place the tip of your tongue against the back of the front teeth, where they meet the roof of your mouth. Just by doing this, you should feel the jaw relax a bit. Welcome to soul lock. That slight movement is the motion that creates it."

"That's it?!" Skye asks incredulously, trying it out himself. Adam nods.

"That's all. It's typical for things that are in the realm of sonship to be easier than we are used to... that's what tends to make them so hard for us to do! Tip of the tongue to the back of the teeth. This is something meant to be applied to *all* your yoga postures, because yoga orphanship brings injury and tension to any of them, and sonship brings the opposite. Just remember to place the tip of the tongue there lightly. If you try really hard you're missing the point. You don't need to do that."

"So what's the indicator that I'm slipping into 'orphanhood' or whatever?" Asks Sylvia.

"Well, after you make the contact, keep your tongue there lightly, and watch to see if your jaw clenches, your tongue starts moving or pressing more firmly into your teeth, or something like that. If these things happen, your effort is too high, either in your mind, body or both."

"Right now, put your tongue in place and try to tense up your jaw. It should be hard to do. The general hope is that if you keep the tongue lightly pressing the teeth, you cannot easily tense up your jaw, so if you do, it means something is off." Aurie raises his hand.

"I was able to do tense my jaw with my tongue there."

"It is possible! But in your practice, if you tense up your jaw, you will probably notice the pressure of the tongue behind the teeth becoming more firm. That's one indicator. If the tongue starts moving around or starts pressing more firmly against the teeth, this is another sign that your effort is outbalancing your ease. Pull back from whatever you're doing in the posture and relax. Yoga orphanship, as we have said, has excess effort that manifests as tension. This very often will manifest as tension in a clenched jaw. I often notice my jaw clenching when I'm in traffic, and have to constantly do soul lock to keep calm cool." You raise your hand quickly.

"What do you mean exactly by excess effort... Too much force or something? I mean, I strive a lot in some poses, and very little in others." You know that time is short, but you have to know. You can see yourself failing the soul lock test in child's pose, but don't understand how anyone could do a pose like this in "yoga orphanship."

"Excess effort means that you are using more effort than you need to be using to complete a certain movement or action. Again, this could be all happening in your mind, body or both. You could be meditating and be using too much effort. I personally think that yoga orphanship almost always starts in the mind and manifests outward to the body. That's what soul lock is all about. It doesn't really bring your body into alignment, but it acts more as a "sonship thermometer" to tell you where you are in your balance of effort and ease. Hopefully, if you're getting out of balance, you notice before you get hurt."

"This means that if you're constantly giving attention to soul lock and you're not able to keep the contact soft and/or light with your tongue, then it's time to back off from the posture and maybe your practice for the day. Just take a break, take some time to find a good modification or find some way of applying less effort. Examine what you were thinking about at the time. You want to find more of a balance between effort and ease and if you fail soul lock, it just isn't happening at that moment. I want you guys to really listen to me for a second... Bella, I know you want to go, but this is really important." Adam steps forward a bit.

"*Listen listen listen!*"

"Feeling excess tension doesn't mean you are acting like an orphan in your practice. *Not adjusting* to balance the tension with ease means you might be. Sonship would be to back off and maybe make a modification to your pose. Orphanship would be to power through it or something like that... That's what leads to injury."

"Okay, I've held you long enough – have a good week all! Next week we start with alignment concepts." You begin to pack up and head home, with thoughts of tongues and orphans dancing through your head.

CHAPTER 6

HEAD, SHOULDERS KNEES & TOES, PART 1

You start this class, fresh and ready, pen in hand and excited to move away from the locks. They have helped your posture quite a bit, but spending too much time on one topic always makes you feel a little "stuck" in slow motion. Adam walks into the room and starts writing on the board.

"Before we get started, lets review the locks." You can barely suppress a groan, and put your pen down. Adam continues. "When you start doing this lock that I am thinking of now, you want to be sure you lift the spine so that it's straight. The head is then pulled back a little while the chin is tucked. Anyone?" You lazily look around, but find only a classroom of people staring at their desks. Finally you raise your hand.

"Throat lock?" you ask hopefully. Adam smiles.

"You got it! Throat lock. The neck is stretched and the chin tucked. As long as the chin is down and the back is straight your are on your way to a good throat lock. This lock is easy to do and full of benefits, so you should be able to use it in most of your postures. You'll do every posture better because of it. Okay, lets get on to today's class." You smile in spite of your earlier annoyance, feeling pretty good about the fact that you're the only one who knew the answer. Adam starts the new material.

"One of the things that's so great about yoga is that it moves and stretches so many parts of our body. That makes it just as good or better than a wide variety of other forms of exercise out there. If you do your posture practice with a relaxed, peaceful, happy disposition, your body will thrive and grow. If you strive and push yourself too much, you may get hurt. Of course, if you don't do anything at all besides watch TV, that's no good either. Generally speaking, one big key to staying young is to keep moving, and yoga is a great daily practice. If you can't do your postures that day, at least take a stroll down the road or around the block! Your body with thank you."

"So… how do we treat our body well in yoga? How do we avoid hurting ourselves in stretches? We talked about soul lock and yoga sonship last week, and there are other principles that are important as well. Lets go over some key terms, which Rhema Yoga calls the 8 Instances. These are things that take place throughout your body while you are moving through your postures and flows. Pay close attention, you'll need to have a complete understanding of each of these terms for the exam." You furrow your eyebrows at this comment. The idea of a final exam for a lecture series that you already paid for still does not excite you. Adam makes the following list on the whiteboard:

Tension & Compression
Movers & Stabilizers
Stability & Mobility
Range of Motion
Core Movement
Contraction
Spiraling
Rotation

"Right then... I'm not going to do this in order... I just wanted to make an upside down triangle with my list." The class chuckles, and that seems to give everyone a bit of an energy boost. Adam underlines an item on the list. "The first instance I want to cover is 'movers and stabilizers.' The meaning is generally pretty clear from the name." Adam takes a thick, black marker that you've never seen before, and writes out a definition on the board:

The instance of "movers and stabilizers" describes the moments when different muscles act as either a mover or a stabilizer in your poses.

"Every muscle you have plays an important roll of both a mover and a stabilizer in your body. Which role a muscle is playing in any one particular moment, however, depends on the exact movement occurring at that time. So you can see how the role of a muscle will switch multiple times throughout your posture practice from mover to stabilizer, back to mover and again to stabilizer, over and over again. During your practice, a muscle acting as a mover helps to initiate movements in all of your postures, and a muscle acting as a stabilizer helps to stabilize the movement. Does that make sense to you all? Seem clear?" You hardly have time to consider his question, scribbling in your notebook as quickly as possible. You guess that the other students are doing the same, because the room is quite except for the sound of pens on paper. Adam continues.

"Good! Lets move on to the next instance, called 'rotation.' Whereas the last term discussed the role of muscles in your postures, this instance specifically pinpoints the movement at a joint in your postures. So…" Again Adam moves to the board to write out a definition.

The instance of "rotation" describes a moment when movement at a joint moves a limb, or part of a limb, towards or away from the frontal midline of the body.

"With that definition in mind, lets start off with internal rotation. Should be easy enough to understand I think. Internal rotation is about the movement which rotates the limb, or a part of a limb, *inwards* towards the medial line of the frontal body." Sylvia raises her hand, and Adam pauses for her.

"What is the front medial line? What's midline?"

"Good question!" Adam answers, hopping back to the his pile of

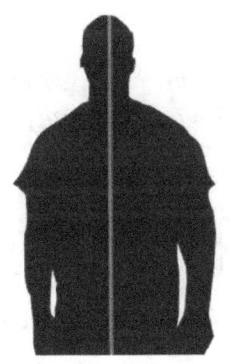

papers to grab a laminated picture. He tapes it up, and it shows the silhouette of a person with a line going right through the middle of his body. "A median line is pretty much what it looks like here; a line through the middle of something. So internal rotation is what brings a part of the body in towards this middle line, but only the middle line in the front of your body, not the back. And since we're on the topic, we might as well go right on ahead towards 'external rotation.' External rotation is a movement at a joint that rotates a limb or some part of a limb, just like internal rotation does. The key difference here is, as you may have already guessed, that you are not bringing a part of your body inward. Instead, you are bringing a part of your body outward and away from the front midline of the body." He points towards the middle line that runs through the man in the picture with one hand, and draws a little arrow pointing away from the line with the other. So this is a basic idea in the realm of alignment that you'll want to understand to some degree now, and to an ever-greater degree as you expand your practice. That is, internal and external rotation in relation to the frontal medial line of the body."

"Okay, spiraling now. I'm not going to go too deep into this next section, because it's really something more for our advanced level students, most who are going for their Rhema Registered Yoga Teacher 500 (R-RYT 500) certification. But it's good to know at least a bit about in case someone references it in a conversation or class you are in."

The instance of "spiraling" describes a moment when your muscle rotates around the bone either inwardly or outwardly, in relation to the front middle of the body.

"As you might guess, an inner spiral is a situation to describe the moment when your muscle rotates around the bone inward, toward the front and centerline of the body. Front centerline is what we are talking about when we are referencing that frontal medial line." He quickly taps the picture again. "So, as you might guess, that makes the outer spiral a time when the muscle rotates around the bone *outward – so it goes* away from the front and centerline of the body. Just like outward rotation is talking about moving a part of your body away from the centerline, so outward spiraling is talking about rotating a muscle away from the centerline. This can be helpful to think about when you're doing your postures, but it really isn't something we talk about too much at these lectures or even at the R-RYT 200 level. Now, lets talk core movement!"

"The core is a popular topic for fitness, sports and general health these days, and it always has been a hot topic in yoga. So… what is it? Any ideas?" The room is generally silent, and you have no idea either. After a second or two, Adam continues.

"The core is a major part of our body, composed of major muscles such as the pelvic floor muscles, the transverses abdominals, the multifidus, the internal and external oblique, the rectus abdominis, the erector spinae and the diaphragm. If you have ever done '3-part breath' with me at any of my classes you have used all of these muscles just by doing that breathing exercise, because your core is involved in everything you do, even breathing! So, going back to our white board of definitions here…"

The instance of "core movement" describes a moment when muscles in the core engage and cause movement. This is especially important when initiating movement.

"There is a small list of minor core muscles as well, and they include the latissimus dorsi, gluteus maximus and the trapezius." Aurie throws his pencil down, almost in disgust.

"I don't know how to even spell those, much less understand where they are or what they do!" You take your concentration off the board and look over to the older man sitting next to you in his familiar black leather. Today he's gone bald, by choice, and shaved all of his hair off. It makes him look a little scary, and definitely highlights the frustration on his face. Adam turns to the board and writes out a quick blurb:

Core: The torso!

For now, just think about all of the muscles in your upper, mid and lower torso… that's what I've basically listed off just now. The major muscles of the core are all somewhere in the area of the belly and the mid and lower back. Please be sure to take note that I'm *not* including the shoulders here! They are not centrally located in your torso and they are not your core."

"Other peripheral areas outside of the core include the hips, shoulders and neck. These are not the core, even though they are important as well. If you ever start teaching about the core, you may need to know more and say more than this. For now, if you can just remember that the core is broadly considered to be the muscles in the torso, and that healthy movement initiates from the core, you'll be fine. Your posture practice should include movements that initiate from your core because as you can imagine, movement is highly dependent on this part of the body. So if you do not initiate your movements from here, they will take more energy to do, and could lead to injury. That's why it's important to exercise your core muscles and learn to initiate posture movement from them."

"If you don't work out your core muscles, that could be a concern as well, even if you are initiating movement from that area. A lack of core muscular development can result in injury too, especially as you progress to some of the more advanced poses in yoga. When it comes to yoga and real life, your core muscles are responsible for initiating most full-body functional movement. They play a large part in determining a person's posture and even their ability to take a deep breath. That's one reason we work out our core so much in 3-part breath, it's all core functionality!" Adam looks over to Aurie. "Does that give you a better idea?" Aurie looks cynical. Almost like he asked what Santa Claus looked like, and Adam had just drawn him a stick figure. Adam sighs.

"Okay, I'll go off lesson plan just this once. Lets dig a bit deeper into the core." He turns to the whiteboard and sketches out a title, which he underlines.

Major Muscles in the Core

"The first muscle we'll discuss is the diaphragm. You all use this every day, all day, because the diaphragm functions in both respiration and stability. As you may know, the diaphragm is responsible for pumping air in and out of the lungs, allowing you to breath. However, it's also the muscle closest to everything else in your core. There's nothing more proximal than the diaphragm. That's why it also helps to stabilize the upper and lower body, which is key in your yoga postures."

"Respiration, or breathing, is needed every second to stay alive, and healthy respiration makes your poses that much more strong and stable. Stability is needed if you want to do anything more than rest on the floor or something, so obviously we're talking about a very important muscle for living, not just doing yoga. Okay... we established that when we do 3-part breath, we are giving the diaphragm a good workout." He sketches out quick notes to everything he's saying as he speaks, and at the end of the last line, turns to the class and takes a quick look at Aurie. "Does that makes sense so far?" Aurie and the rest of the class nod, and Adam turns back to the board.

"Okay cool! We're making progress. Let's jump on over from the diaphragm to the abdominal muscles then. The abdominal muscles, or abs, include several of the confusing names I listed off earlier. They are the transverses abdominals, internal and external oblique's and rectus abdominals. When you think abs, think these four. In terms of what they do and why they are important to Rhema Yoga, the reason is the same. All of these muscles are primary core stabilizers, and all of them are used during inhalation and exhalation. So, as you can imagine, 3-part breath exercises all of the abs as well. One of the themes you'll see as I dig deeper into the core is that 3-part breath and the core are buddies; you can't really talk about one without eventually discussing the other. Alright... lets move on to the pelvic floor then."

"The pelvic floor muscles play a huge role in inhalation and exhalation, believe it or not. I was shocked to hear it, because I never think of that area as a component of my breath. But it is indeed! If the diaphragm is the top muscle that stimulates breath, the pelvic floor is the bottom. Almost like the diaphragm is the top of your 'air container' and the pelvic floor is the bottom of that container. They work together in each breath you take."

"That being the case, it might not surprise you to hear that the pelvic floor can be called the pelvic diaphragm as well. It is a key muscle of the core container, and our 3-part breath exercises these muscles well." He stops then, and decides to dive into his bag for something. The class sits in silence for a minute or two before Adam stands up again and tapes the following picture to the board. "This," he says, pointing to the picture nearby, is called the multifidus muscle, which we'll talk about next."

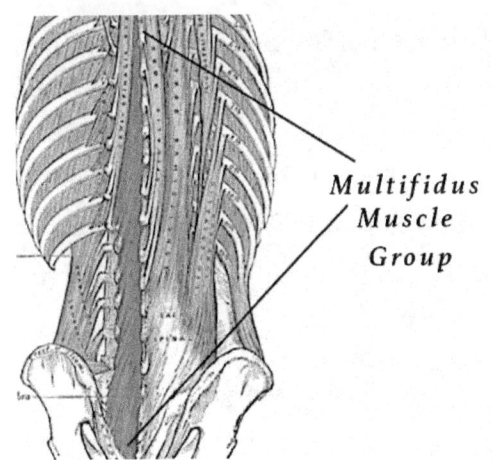

Multifidus
Muscle
Group

"The multifidus muscle is actually a very thin, somewhat small muscle. On the picture here, it looks like one big muscle that goes all the way up your back, but that's not really the case. It sits deep in the spine and only spans about three joint segments. So the picture is actually made up of a lot of small, segmental muscles. They run the entire length of your spine, all the way from your pelvis to the highest vertebra of your neck. From there, each one works to stabilize your joints at a segmental level. This muscle is pretty stiff and stable, and that helps each vertebra work more effectively, slowing down the degeneration of the joints. As you can imagine, it's a big muscle group with a serious role to play! Still, I'll bet that until today, most of you have never heard of it. This is a really deep back muscle so for the most part, it's covered by larger muscles. Don't take it for granted though because this thin muscle still plays an important role in stabilizing the spine. I usually don't talk about it too much for the 'Stretchers' class, so if you want to know more, take my 'Yog(a)natomy' class, or buy the book. We're going to move on now, to quickly cover the Erector Spinea." He starts a sudden, frantic search through his bag again, and pulls out another picture for the whiteboard within a few seconds. At this point, the whiteboard is almost completely covered with pictures and writing, but it makes you happy to see a teacher trying so hard. Adam points to his newest picture, now hanging from the corner of the whiteboard.

"This set of three muscles, called spinal erectors, work together to create an extension of the vertebral column. This is what gives you

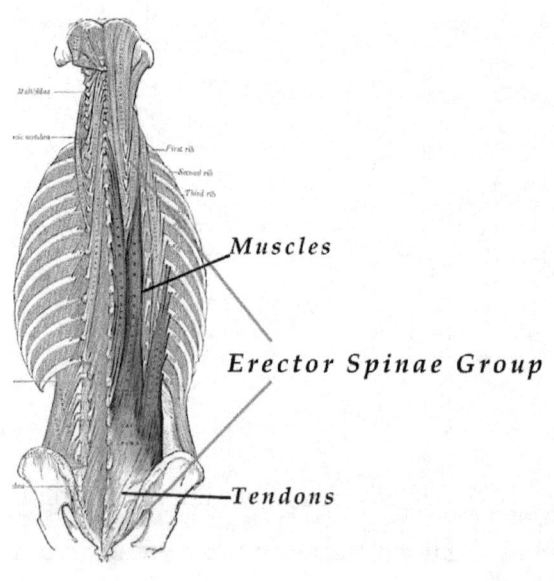

that erect posture, straightening out your back. When you rotate the back in a side-to-side movement, you're also engaging these. They sit on each side of the vertebral column and extend alongside almost the entire spine, including our three favorite curves. Anyone able to rattle them off for us?" Skye almost jumps out of his chair.

"Lumbar, thoracic and cervical!" Adam laughs.

"You got it. All three major sections of the spine. If you injure or strain this muscle you'll know it quickly, because it often results in back spasms and a lot of pain. One last thing. When you think about the erector spinae, remember that they are not just one muscle, but a bundle of muscles and tendons working together." He puts his marker down.

"There's really no need to dig deeper into them for this class, or the other minor core muscles. I'll just say that the minor core muscles are the latissimus dorsi, gluteus maximus, and the trapezius. Good ol' 3-part exercises the latissumus dorsi and the trapezius muscles as well, but not the gluts." Adam glances to the clock quickly and lets out a quick gasp.

"Oh man! We're really behind schedule! Okay, let me go ahead, we need to move fast to cover everything!" He finds a clean piece of whiteboard, and starts writing.

The instance of "contraction" describes a moment when your muscles are activated either concentrically or eccentrically, isometrically or isotonically.

"From the core movement, we're going to go to muscle contraction. As you might guess, your muscles are constantly contracting when you are doing your posture practice, and there are two types of contraction that we will define now. The first is concentric contraction, which is a case of your muscle being shortened and contracted. The second is eccentric contraction, a time when your muscle is lengthened and contracted. One is not more important or better than the other in your practice. For now, it's good enough for you to know about and understand the terms. A muscle is made strong and healthy when it is regularly concentrically and eccentrically contracted, and that is what our posture practice is full of. So as you can guess, and probably already knew, a regular posture practice is very good for your muscles. It features regular concentric and eccentric contraction. Another important topic for us to review is tension and compression."

The instance of "tension and compression" describes a moment when range of motion is stopped because of limitations in either the muscle or bone.

"This was huge for me when I was first learning how far to push myself in postures. It also gave me a lot of hope for poses that I thought would never be able to do because I just wasn't flexible enough." Bella raises her hand, but Adam seems on a mission since glimpsing the clock. "Sorry Bella, let me get into this or I might forget what I want to say here." She nods, but he has already turned to the whiteboard again. "When a muscle is stretched to its maximum ability, further movement is inhibited by tension. For me, when I was first learning yoga and unable to get my heels to the floor in downward facing dog, this was the case. My hamstrings were stretched as far as they were willing to go, and the tension in my muscles let me know that I wasn't safely going any further. I thought that this meant I would never get my heels to the floor, but I found out later that the more I did yoga, the farther I could stretch my hamstrings before that tension stopped me. That was a good day indeed! It meant that I just needed to slowly build up the flexibility and strength in my legs."

"Sometimes however, further movement is inhibited due to bone structure. In this case, it's not muscles stopping you, but bone meeting bone that is creating compression. If you sense that happening, you're done, and really need to respect what your body is trying to tell you. If I was in downward facing dog and unable to get my heels to the floor because of compression, that would be it for my range of motion in down-dog. So, it is possible to move further into a pose that is currently inhibited by muscle tension, but any movement past compression will not occur, and can definitely lead to injury if you push too hard. Now, once again, tension shouldn't be ignored in your yoga pose! You need to respect your muscles if they give you tension that tells you to stop! If you act like a yoga orphan you'll push past that tension and end up straining muscles, or worse. Act like a yoga son or daughter and respect your body, celebrating whatever progress you can get that day. Remember, our posture practice is about body worship to God, not really anything else." He stops here, pulls out a bottle of water from his bag, and takes a big swig.

"Phew! I can tell we're trying to cover a lot today, I'm chatting up a storm. Don't' worry too much if you miss something – you can always ask questions on our online class page, or talk to me directly outside of class hours." He puts his bottle down, picks his marker up, and begins writing again.

"Next is 'range of motion.' This range of motion is in relation to motion as it applies to the body. So it's the range at which a joint can move both easily and easefully, without needing help from other muscles."

The instance called "range of motion" describes the moments when a joint moves easily and freely in a posture practice, without needing help from other muscles.

"If a joint has to start enlisting other muscles that normally or ideally would be unnecessary, just to complete its range of motion, this will cause tension elsewhere in the body or in the joint itself. So if you're having tension when you're trying to increase your range of motion, it's because your joints are too weak or limited to do what you're asking them to do, and they're drafting the help of other muscles that are nearby. This might seem like a confusing instance, because the term 'range of motion' is actually noun, describing the range. However, we decided to use it because it is a common term in the physical therapy and yoga world, and it is used the same way there. Okay, so that's range of motion. Now we move on to the relationship, or partnership, of stability and mobility. Got your pens ready?"

The instance called "stability and mobility" describes the moments when you are either stable or mobile in your practice.

Stability is dependent on mobility. It comes from the effort needed to contract some muscles while releasing others. When you can do it in a way that balances the energy you are expending in different parts of your body, you are stable. Mobility is the body's ability to partake in all of the various posture movements with ease in both connective and muscle tissue. We all want to increase our mobility, which is one reason we do yoga, so mobility and stability are good to know about and keep in mind." Adam takes a deep breath, chugs his water one last time, and looks back at the whiteboard.

"Well, we covered a lot more than I thought we would, but we're a bit behind schedule because of our talk about the core. Next week we'll pick up from here and finish talking about alignment and the main parts of the body. We don't have any time for questions now, but just send a message to our class page if you want to discuss anything – good job all, we had a busy day!" Sylvia, the girl in front of you, finishes off her bottle of grape soda and starts to pack up, and you decide to do the same.

CHAPTER 7

HEAD, SHOULDERS KNEES & TOES, PART 2

You come to class on time today and take your usual seat, a little groggy and nursing a headache from what has already been a hard day of work at the office. Adam enters the class a bit late, and seems hurried. "Well, these next two classes are times that I build into the schedule with the idea that we'll be behind in our material and will need cover whatever is left in order to take the midterm test, so we're okay… but lets hit the ground running. We did the 8 Instances, but I'm about to hit you with another list, because our class topic today will introduce to you what I call the 7 Stars. These are different than our list yesterday, and they are just important for your postures, if not more, because the stars point out key areas of the body. We will describe their basic function, and then discuss how this function relates to your posture practice. The Instances, in contrast, describe things that happen in different areas of your body while you do your poses. Here in the 7 Stars, we have what we call the abdominal core, or ab core. Don't confuse that with core movement, which we discussed last week with the Instances. The ab core focuses on only a specific part of your core. It talks about what happens in that part of core." Adam seems satisfied with his explanation, and takes a bunch of dry-erase markers from his bag. He turns to the board and starts writing in blue ink:

The Feet

"As with the muscle locks, we're going to start our discussion of the 7 stars from the bottom and move up. Just as we discussed with foot lock, the main role of your feet in your posture practice is to support the entire body. Your feet are the foundation for all standing poses, but there's more to say on how they do that, and what it looks like when they do it well. When you are healthy and engaged from the bottom up, your feet provide a dynamic foundation that flexes, strengthens and softens with every pose. In our world off the mat and outside of class, it is our feet that allow us to stand, walk, run and get all that stability and mobility. As you might guess, the feet are a big deal! They are active in all inversions and arm balances, most backbends, forward bends, and many twists and hip openers." Sylvia raises her hand.

"Inversions? What are they? Is that something we do?"

"Oh! Right, sorry... good question! So an inversion is a pose in which you sort of 'go upside down,' if that makes sense. Your heart is over your head. Typical inversions include postures like shoulder stand, headstand, handstand and forearm stand. Inversions almost always strengthen the arms, legs, back and core abdominal muscles. Does that make sense?" Sylvia nods, and Adam continues.

"Again, the feet are pretty important parts of your body – don't take them for granted or overlook them! So many people do. We'd all be much better off if we provided a little lovin' to our feet now and again. That's one reason many Rhema Yoga sequences start off with foot work! Our feet provide all that stability, mobility and support we mentioned, while at the same time being consistently subject to stress. One of the primarily stressors for our feet comes from shoes, believe it or not. High heels are particularly nasty. A serious lack of strength and flexibility is what we get from wearing shoes. Of couse we need to wear them, but it's worth it to buy good ones, and to love your feet well with different exercises. Lack in strength and flexibility is what contributes to a deficiency in our balance. Both our balance and our success at a healthy posture are in jeopardy when we don't love our feet well." You raise your hand cautiously.

"What do you mean when you say 'love our feet well?' What does that look like?"

"Well, there are a lot of things you can do, and in other lectures we teach you how. For now, I'll just say that it's pretty important to do things that increase strength, flexibility and resilience in the foot. That's where yoga in general comes in and helps out. Even practicing foot lock helps to improve the health of the feet, and subsequently the function of our whole body. Like I said, get good shoes; pay a little bit of extra money for the better pair. Then, learn about and try some of the other things we do in Rhema to improve our foot health. All of these things come together to aid with both our practice and our daily life." Adam grabs his blue marker again and begins writing another item on his list.

The Knees

"Moving up from the feet, we have the knees, which are primarily intended to extend and flex. This is what they do when we walk, run, sit, or anything else. Are you with me so far about extension and flexion?" There is silence, and blank stares. Adam laughs. "I can't tell if you're confused or just bored. Well, extension in the knee constitutes movement from a bent-knee position to a straight-leg position, right? So if you were kicking a ball, that would be extension. Knee flexion is different. It's a case of you curling your leg back, like if you were going to kick yourself in the butt with the bottom of your foot. Your heel goes up, toward the ceiling. Okay?" More silence, so Adam goes on. "In a way it's good you are all so quiet, because we have a lot of ground yet to cover if we're going to be ready for the midterm in a few weeks!"

"Now, I want you to be sure that you understand and remember what I'm about to say next; the knees can extend and flex very well, but they have only minor capability for any sort of rotating motion. They are built to extend and flex, not rotate. You'll want to keep in mind that a sudden or excessive movement in any direction can tear one of the knee's supporting ligaments, tendons or cartilage – no matter what that movement is – but rotation is by far the riskiest! When you begin asking the knee to participate in something that it's not really meant to do too much of, use caution. Avoid it if possible." He puts up an picture of the knee on the white board. "As you can see from all the tendons and ligaments here in the picture, there is a lot of mobility and motion built into the knee. Yet so many yogis, runners and other athletes, as well as those with a consistent meditation practice, all repeatedly discover how painful it can be to damage their ligaments and tendons. They often ask their knees to do things that they are simply not meant to do, and the stress created from such activities lead to incapacitating injury." Adam stops, adjusts his marker, and taps on the picture of the knee.

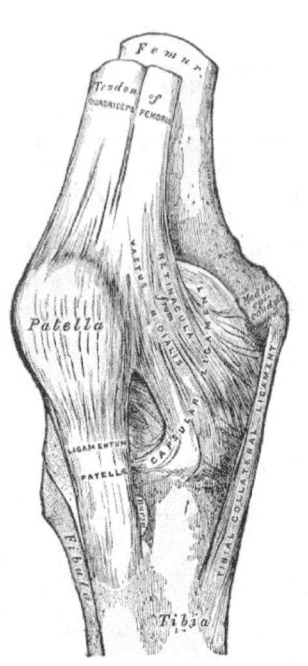

"Remember! Knee injury is most frequently going to be in the tendons, ligaments or cartilage – all of those things that allow for flex and extend actions. Because these parts of the knee receive less blood supply than the muscles, they almost always take longer to heal than muscle injuries too. Anything that receives less blood almost always takes longer to heal and has a greater likelihood for injury. The good news is that understanding the basic functional capacity of the knee can reduce and maybe even eliminate potential for injury in your yoga practice. It doesn't matter whether you are doing postures, meditation, breathing or something else."

"So then, because the knee is so important, lets talk a bit about how to keep it healthy. We'll use what I call the 'Big 3' for healthy knees. Let me write them out:"

The Big 3
Provide Stability – Prevent Strain – Maintain Alignment.

"If you keep the Big 3 in mind, you'll go a long way in maintaining healthy, happy knees throughout your practice and in your everyday life. As you might have noticed by now, and as I keep saying, so many things we do on the mat translate to our everyday lives, and this is one of them too. Get your pen and paper out and get ready, because we're going to talk about what the Big 3 is, and how to do it. Ready?" The class is silent, so Adam takes a new part of the board to write sketches out a title.

Start with Stability

"The key indicator for a stable knee is in the kneecap. You'll know your knee joint is stabilized when you cannot move the kneecap from side to side with your hand. If you try to move your kneecap now, when you muscles are not flexed, you'll notice a fair amount of movement is possible. Engaging the quadriceps muscles, or 'quads,' puts a stop to that almost immediately. Flexing the quads is the most important action to take in creating the stability you want in your knee. In case you've forgotten what the quads are, or never really knew, I'll tell you now."

"When you think 'quads,' think about the large muscles that are in the front of your legs, above your knee. Your quads are actually a muscle group, although most people think of them as only one or two muscles. In reality, there are four! They are the Rectus Femoris, which is the muscle in the middle and front of your thigh, the Vastus Intermedius, which sits nestled behind the Rectus Femoris, the Vastus Lateralis, which is on the side of your thigh, and the Vastus Medialis, which sits on the inner thigh. You don't have to remember the names of these muscles, or even where they are, but you do want to remember that the quad is a group of four muscles. You also want to remember where this muscle group is, and that it stabilizes your knee."

"Other than the quads, engaging the back and inner thigh is another ideal action to take if you want to stabilize the knee. This is something you would do whenever the knees are straight and bearing weight. When might that happen?"

"When you're standing up" Bella says, almost without thinking.

"Right you are Bella! So when you're in a standing pose, you'll want to remember to engage both quads and thighs. Actually, when you are in your standing poses, you are engaging both your foot and leg muscles, so these postures are very active for your lower body, if

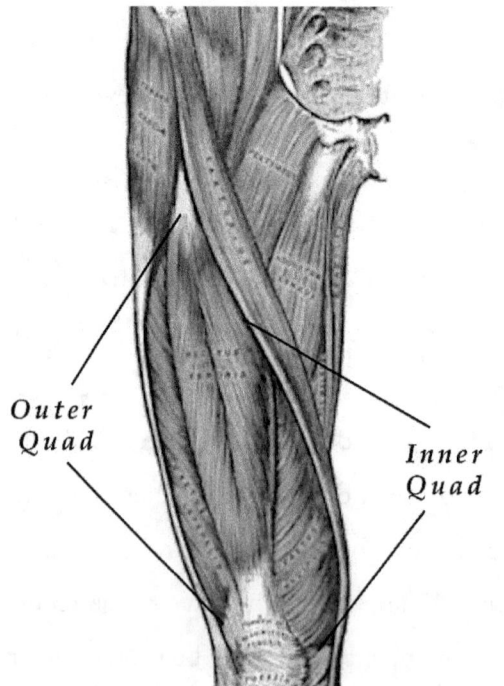

Outer Quad

Inner Quad

nowhere else. Remember that in standing poses, everything begins with the feet and travels up to the knee, first and foremost." Bella raises her hand.

"So is this knee lock or something?" Adam shakes his head.

"I know what you're thinking, because I asked the exact same question when I was learning about all of this. There isn't a knee lock. Even though you are engaging muscles to keep your kneecap from sliding, you are not locking your knee. So *stabilizing* the knee and *locking* the knee are two very different things. It's not that you'll have a huge problem or health risk if you do lock you knee, but you want to avoid it more times than not because when you lock your knee, your actually pushing your knee to its maximum possible extension. When the knees are extended to their maximum, you're losing some strength and flexibility and becoming a bit more rigid. Also, it's really difficult to engage all of the other leg muscles you may need for your poses. So we don't 'lock' the knee if we can help it. The focus is to stabilize, and stabilizing actions come from your quads, both inner and outer. If you work on strengthening both of them in a balanced way, you'll promote long-term support for two healthy knees. Not only that, you'll also be able to easily engage the other muscles in your leg as needed while in your standing poses. This will make your poses more aligned, easier to do, and more rewarding in the long run. Okay, that's enough on stabilizing, lets move on to strain." Adam writes it on the board before continuing.

Secondly, Strain

"Here is where the idea of yoga sonship and a little bit of knowledge can save you a lot of pain. In yoga, there are some poses, such as hero and half hero, where your knees will be flexed to their maximum. This in not a problem if your focus is on stretching the leg and hip muscles, *not* the ligaments around the knee. Again, we're talking about loving your knee and taking care of your ligaments and tendons. Too many people stretch their ligaments, not their muscles, and pay a price. Sharp pains in the knees are your clear warning that something needs to be modified right away. If you are unable to find a good modification, you might want to just come out of the pose you're trying to do. Even mild pain on the inside or outside of the knee is a signal for you to modify or come out." Bella raises her hand again.

"What about just a small stretching sensation or something. I get that a lot... it doesn't hurt, but I can tell something is happening and it feels like a... like a sort of stretch. Is that okay?"

"Yes, generally that's fine. Just watch it and be sure it doesn't change into pain. Sometimes, when we don't feel pain in our knees while we are doing a pose, we stop paying attention to them. A few moments later when our knees start to hurt we are slow to recognize it, because we are so busy focusing on other things in our body. Remember that your tendons and ligaments heal a lot less quickly than your muscles, so if you make a mistake, it may take a while to recover. It's worth it to monitor your knees as you do your poses, and take it slow and easy all the way through. Also, be prop friendly! I mentioned hero pose just now. When you're doing that, you may want to raise your butt up a bit with blankets or a block. Things like that go a long way in helping you care for your body while still getting a good stretch. I know that when I'm in child's pose, placing a rolled up blanket as far into the knee pit as possible before actually bending the knee can relieve a lot of pressure for them." He turns back to his list on the board:

Finally, Alignment

"Last but not least, the Big 3 finishes off with concerns about alignment. When it comes to knee positioning, you need to remember to keep your knees in line with your toes at all times. It doesn't matter if you're in bridge, mountain, warrior 2 or warrior 1. You could be in vogue pose, wheel pose, or any other pose. This concept always remains the same. Often it will just happen naturally because your body wants to be aligned, especially in the area of knees and toes, but there will also be times when you'll need to pay attention and make adjustments. This is especially true for anyone who has spent some time training their body on how to do certain poses in the other systems of yoga. Although famous and popular, these systems are not necessarily made for modern American bodies, and could create habits in some poses that do not encourage alignment or OSP."

"Alright, I think I've covered the knees for now, lets move on... that clock keeps ticking and we still have a lot to discuss! Moving up from the feet and then the knee, we come to the third star, the pelvis." Adam moves to the board again, adding to the list. At this point there are indeed three items written down.

The Foot

The Knee

The Pelvis

"When it comes to the pelvis, one thing you'll want to consider quite a bit is positioning. The position of the pelvis will determine much about the alignment of the spine, and primarily the lumbar spine. What part of the spine is the lumbar spine?" Skye, who had been writing like a maniac in his notes so far, quickly raises his hand.

"The lower back, below the thoracic!"

"Good!" Adam says, giving him a quick thumbs up. Aurie whispers something hostile under his breath, but you can't make it out.

"So, the lumbar spine and the pelvis are pretty close together and they affect each other quite a bit. Don't forget though, the rest of the spine will be affected by the position of the pelvis as well. Earlier in this workshop series we spoke about how the other curves are affected when one curve moves more in or out of it's natural state, do you remember? When the pelvis affects the lumbar, the thoracic and cervical are affected as well in a sort of domino affect."

"This being true, one can see clearly that if pelvis is at neutral, the spine may more easily come into its natural curvature. The problem is that most people have a tendency to tilt their pelvis forward or backward in both their practice and their everyday life. This habitual tilt forward or backward doesn't do our bodies any favors. Tilting acts to either compress or over-stretch the lumbar, tighten the hip flexor muscles, and weaken the abs. That's a lot of negative impact for one small tilt! I have seen some modern yoga systems actually promote a lifestyle of scooping the tailbone under and tilting the pelvis, and over time the result has been a loss of the lumbar curve altogether! Not a good thing."

"In Rhema Yoga, one of the things we do is promote pelvis neutrality in vertical positions. So in plain English, that means that when we are in an upright standing pose or a straight inversion, a neutral pelvis is a goal of ours. It keeps our spine curving in all the right ways and helps us maintain a stable, healthy posture. Again, this absolutely translates off the mat, whether we are walking or standing in place." Adam steps away from the board now, and stands in front of his desk so everyone can see him. Taking his marker, he turns to the side and points it to his hip.

"So look... By stacking the hips over the ankles while lightly applying ab lock, you can create a neutral pelvis, and that allows the spine to find it's natural curves. When you're back bending, you want to remember this because it's important to keep the pelvis neutral in backbends as well. When you remember to keep a neutral pelvis in backbends, you are moving in a way so as *not* to flatten the low back, or lumbar. This contradicts many traditional systems who that give you cues in poses like bridge that will flatten the lumbar. We respectfully disagree with such cues. It might not seem obvious, but if you end up tilting the pelvis and flattening the lumbar, you inhibit movement of the mid and upper back. When that happens, you lose all of the benefits that backbends were designed to give you!"

"Wait wait wait!" Bella says, seemingly without knowing she has. Her face turns red, but she pushes on. "Can you make it clear here? When do we keep the pelvis in neutral and when do we move it away from neutral? I thought it was only neutral in vertical postures like standing poses and some inversions... but you were just talking about backbends too!" Adam nods.

"Good point Bella." He turns back to the board and starts writing again with his trusty blue marker.

When to Move the Pelvis out of Neutral

"It might be easier if we talk about this – situations when a neutral pelvis isn't what you want. This might be easier to understand." He continues writing. "First, whenever you are folding forward while standing – like for forward bends. In this case, if you want to round the low back, the pelvis needs to tip back, and that's fine. You still need to do this in a healthy way, but it's perfectly healthy and good for your fold forward." He turns back to the class. Folding forward with a rounded spine is a poor idea if you have a herniated disk though, so don't go off and start folding like a crazy person if you have disk issues. Maybe come chat with me first. You'll want to tell your students that as well."

"With me so far?" Bella and Skye nod, and you follow their lead. "Okay good. Next, if you want to fold forward at the hips while sitting, and get more stretch in the back of the legs, the pelvis needs to tip forward. Once again, this is fine, and it's actually a good thing, because your really getting a nice stretch for your hamstrings. These forward folds are the two biggest moments when you will not be going for a neutral pelvis position. Okay?" Everyone seems content, so Adam erases a section of whiteboard and moves on.

"The next star is…"

The Ab Core

"Wait, we already talked about the core last week." Aurie points out, lifting his notebook with one hand and raising his other at the same time. Adam turns towards the class.

"Bear with me here, we don't have much time left, and I have to cover all this today. We can chat later if you're still confused." Aurie puts his notebook back on the desk, and Adam turns back to the board. When he is done, he spins back around to the class and starts teaching.

"Strong, toned muscles at the core of the body are super-important for healthy function and posture. We want our core to have powerful muscles that both fuel us and anchor us at the same time. Rhema Yoga poses focus on training our core to act as a stable base as well as a fluid source of movement. Not every sequence we have specifically focuses on the core muscles, but every sequence definitely will have stretches that work them and strengthen them. Ideally, the abdominal muscles are used often and are well toned, but not tense. You want them to be strong as well as sensitive. It's that delicate balance of soft yet strong, sensitive yet forceful. Sometimes people in the gym put too much focus on strengthening their abs and not enough attention on releasing them. This brings a classic imbalance of the body, and inhibits healthy movement. Their abs might look amazing, but they aren't necessarily at a point of maximum health. This is because of a simple concept. When such people focus on strengthening the abs, it often involves a lot of concentric contractions, but not a lot of eccentric contractions. Yoga is wonderful in that it gives your abs a balanced, healthy workout full of the concentric and eccentric contractions that they need."

"I want to stop now and give you all a quick list of things you can do in different poses to focus on your abs. Before I do, I should tell you that you may not be able to remember this list, but it's good to write down and practice from time to time. Maybe just work on these things specifically once in awhile. After some time, you will probably start to do a lot of them automatically."

"First, to tone and strengthen your abdominal core, practice root lock in all the active postures that you do. During your normal posture practice, you are probably not focusing on this, but you might focus on it to a larger degree than normal from time to time. Another thing you can do is practice having a strong focus on drawing the belly button towards the spine during your exhalation."

"When you are working on toning and strengthening your ab core, try to remember that it's important to maintain sensitivity as well. That means that you make sure to include time for softening and relaxing the belly when you're doing your poses. Also, remember to stretch the ab muscles, don't ignore that aspect – they're muscles, and just like every other muscle they need to be stretched! You might be surprised to hear this, but full ab lock can play a large role in helping you with all of these little exercises. It's a great lock for raising awareness in your mind and increasing your 'ab education,' so to speak. Full ab lock's intention is to bring vitality to the core of the body, and as you do it, you will learn more about how your ab core works, different sensations you feel with different actions, and more."

"I'm not sure if you see a difference in the 'star' of 'ab core' vs. the 'instance' of the core movement, but if you don't let me know later. Basically, we're just focusing on a specific area and function of our core here when we discuss the ab core." Adam looks up at the clock and sighs.

"We didn't cover all I wanted to today, but this is as good as a spot to stop at as any. Let's wrap up here and meet next week." He walks over to the lights, dimming them a bit before turning back to the class. "Before we go, how about a 10-minute meditation session just to relax and calm the mind after everything we covered." You put your books away and sit up, happy to focus on the breath and nothing more for a short time.

CHAPTER 7

HEAD, SHOULDERS KNEES & TOES, PART 3

Class starts right on time today, with Adam re-writing his list of four stars from last week before anyone has even come into the room and taken their seat. When everyone has settled in, he looks down at his notes and adds another "star" with red ink, expanding the list to five.

The Spine

"Alrighty then… moving right along to the spine. This is a big one with a lot we could say about it, but remember, we're just going to go with high level information in this lecture. The foundational stuff."

"The spine is designed to be a base for balance and fluidity in your movement, both on and off the mat. It is inherently stable and mobile, but we often mistreat it or ignore it, making it a common place of injury and dis-*ease*. In yoga, one major reason we hurt our spine has to do with yoga orphanship. Many of us, even those of us who have been doing Rhema for awhile, have a tendency to move with force rather than relaxing into the inner intelligence of the soul and body. On top of that, we often like to 'hang' or push into the more mobile parts of the spine – maybe because it feels good or looks good. Maybe simply because we don't know any better. When we do this, we are causing these mobile areas of our spine to become more mobile. The problem is that while we are doing that, other areas become tighter, especially if we ignore them altogether because we are working on our more mobile spots. All of this reduces the original balance of the spine's design and functionality. Things go wrong from here, and injury or dis-ease are almost inevitable if we don't make any changes." Adam takes a deep breath, makes a small hop to his desk to chug some water, and hops back to his place next to the whiteboard.

"Let me try to itemize this out a little for you. You may or may not do these three things I'm about to write, but if you teach, you will almost surely find your students doing them in their postures. A lot of students are operating in yoga orphanship, but a lot of them are also simply taught incorrectly. It's a terrible combination! I call it the 'Evil Twins!' Oh, that will be on your test by the way… I know we didn't talk about it much, but write it down and keep it in your memory! The evil twins are as follows: yoga orphanship and incorrect teaching! Got it?" You scribble it down in a corner of your page, not sure where to put it because it doesn't really flow with anything he's been covering so far.

"Okay good! So, moving on then, I was itemizing. The first thing you'll see is a jutting out of the lower ribs, and a corresponding jamming of the lower back. This will happen most often when students are attempting to open their chest or move into a backward bend. Keep that in mind whenever you give cues around opening the chest or transitioning into back bends. Look at those trouble spots! They are good assisting and adjusting opportunities."

"Second, you're really going to want to watch their pelvis. We talked about this so much already, and the reason is because it's such an issue. Students will often tuck the pelvis and flatten out the lower back, or lumbar, when they are in seated poses or bends. This is very common and, as I mentioned, there are even systems of yoga out there that teach this as one of their main points of instruction! So I blame this on the evil twins, and I'll try my best to remind you to look for it."

"Finally, look for students who hinge at the lower neck when they are looking up or back in their poses. This is a horrible idea, and almost always takes away a good stretch from the student while adding excessive tension. No hinging at the lower neck when your students are looking up or back! The base of the skull goes back, and students can hinge higher up where the spine meets the base of the skull. These are all fine, but hinging at the lower neck is not. Remember that it's not about moving as far as possible in the pose. Poses that want you to look up tend to cause tension – better not to. Look in the same direction that your chest is facing. I know you can see people on social media looking up, and many people love to look up from the lower neck, but in Rhema Yoga, we don't do it."

"Another thing you're going to want to keep in mind is that it can be much harder to rotate at the thoracic spine than in the cervical. We mentioned this earlier. This is because the rib cage is attached to the thoracic, and sort of sits there in the way. As a result, you'll see that many people don't rotate too much in their thoracic, to their own loss. The thoracic is where you get the most reward when you twist and bend. Building on that, make sure that your students don't use their arms to leverage, or basically force the spine to twist too far or over-extend. Especially in the lower back area – this is where many people twist and bend more than they should. They will almost surely hurt themselves sooner or later."

"The reason that students move this way, outside of the evil twins, is because of current posture habits that they have in their everyday lives. We talked about this earlier when we discussed FHS and OSP. Students have FHS and other bad posture patterns that they then bring with them to class, repeating them in their movements and poses. Again, whatever happens on the mat almost always happens off the mat, and vice versa. The repetition of the same imbalanced postures and movements take their toll on the spine. Bad posture and incorrect movement in both everyday life and in our yoga poses results in more permanent imbalances, and these lead to injury later on. Backbends are meant to counter bad posture patterns like FHS and, if they are done correctly, that's exactly what they do. This is why people often say that backbends 'solve everything.'"

"One of the keys then, is alignment of the spine. Remember the "S" shape that we discussed before?" Adam pulls out your corrected drawing from an earlier class and tapes it to the board again. When one part of the spine goes more into it's natural curve, other parts go away from their natural curve. This is how the spine stays balanced, and it's beautiful in design. Habitual mis-use, however, can and will lead to painful times!"

"To prevent straining the muscles and tissue around the spine, remember to draw muscular energy toward the core and lead movements from there. This helps when you are trying to find good posture, and it also helps you stay away from an attitude of yoga orphanship that you might bring to your yoga practice, complete with overstretching and overworking" Aurie can't help himself and starts raising his hand, but Adam keeps talking, although he does point at Aurie, almost as if he is guessing the question. "Drawing muscular energy toward the core might seem too abstract to be practical advice, but remember that we can do it easily – this is not metaphysical mumbo-jumbo! Practice your locks! Root lock and ab lock. Don't forget other core strengthening exercises either. These will all do the job. Actually, 3-part breath and the muscle locks are very helpful here." He suddenly taps the board a few times, and you guess that it's to make sure everyone is awake and paying attention.

"So! To maintain a healthy alignment of the spine, we want to move the spine regularly in all directions. This means we need a yoga practice complete with forward bends, backward bends, side bends and twists. Almost every sequence should have at least some of these. Also, remember to focus on gently cultivating flexibility in the less mobile parts of the spine, such as the lumbar, which is the least mobile part of the three we discussed. The thoracic spine can twist more, and it actually needs to twist more than the lumbar spine, so use leverage to get a good twist in your thoracic. Finally, and this goes back to our talks in earlier classes, remember to fight FHS with OSP. Focus on countering any habitual, dysfunctional postures and movements you see by using what we learned."

"This sort of basic, foundational knowledge about the spine and your posture is what 'Stretchers' is all about. The 4 Legs of Rhema Yoga become *much* more rewarding if you remember and apply the basics. That's why we're here." Adam smiles, looking proud of himself for a moment. He starts moving again when he glances at the clock. "Gosh, we are *late late late!* I really need to make this workshop series a week or two longer." You silently thank your lucky starts that you signed up for the classes now, in case he extends it to another 1-2 weeks later, and Adam adds another item to his list. When he turns back to the class, it looks like this:

The Foot

The Knee

The Pelvis

The Ab Core

The Spine

The Wrists

"Since wrist pain is a common complaint in yoga postures, this is an important star. Sometimes your student will approach you about wrist pain, and it will be because they spend long hours on the computer, or doing other activities throughout their day that inflame it. That said, wrist pain can also be a common result of postures and stretches. My teacher told us that awhile ago yoga instructors always informed students that if they have wrist pain, it was never because of the yoga. Now, we know that is not necessarily the case. Whether the problem of wrist pain begins in your class or in your life, bearing weight in the hands in different yoga postures can exacerbate it. Fortunately, bearing weight in the hands the right way during your yoga class can also prevent future damage and be the needed therapy for current pain. Hard to believe, huh? The answer lies in knowing how to approach the issue skillfully."

"First of all, lets talk full wrist extension. Adam sees a little confusion in the room, so he is quick to add that "Full wrist extension is a 90-degree angle between the hand and forearm. A lack of full, healthy wrist movement is why most people gradually lose the ability to move easily and safely into full wrist extension. That's a big deal because dynamic yoga practices require this position of the wrist in many postures. Examples anyone?"

"Handstand?" Skye asks?

"Right you are Skye! Good! Plank, low plank, and arm balances like crow pose all require a good, strong wrist extension. In order to prevent a straining in the wrists from overstretching or overworking in these poses, it's important to recognize the potential need to work up weight-bearing capability in the wrists and in the hands. It's okay to do that slowly, too. This really isn't a race. Just be sure to distribute the weight into the front of the palm and in the inner heel while drawing up through the wrists and arms, that's hand lock, which we covered earlier. Hand lock really does save the wrists. I know I said it before when we covered locks, but I really want you to remember it. This lock and star really do go hand-in-hand, so to speak. Okay, lets finish these off!"

The Shoulders

The shoulder is a ball and socket joint, and it's designed to offer an extreme range of motion. Compared to other joints, nothing really comes too close to the mobility you'll find in your shoulders. This is because the socket is more shallow than similar ball and socket joints like the hips. Of course, these days a lot of that mobility has become quite diminished for a large number of people. The reason, once again, lies in daily life. The habitual repetition of daily activities such as driving, working on a computer, sitting on the couch and habitually slouching the shoulders forward all work to degrade shoulder mobility. Our shoulders are designed to have a huge range of motion, but if you don't use it you lose it."

"What's more, that extreme range of motion that is offered to you in your shoulders can be a double-edged sword. A greater range of motion comes with a much greater risk of injury. I just said that the shoulder socket is very shallow. Because of that, it's all the more important to remember that when you approach movement and use of the shoulders in your practice, you focus on stability and mobility. The best way to prevent strain while you build and maintain healthy function of the shoulder joints is to *find a balance between shoulder stability and shoulder mobility in all of your postures.* That's the key." Sylvia raises her hand.

"How to be stable? What do you need to do? Is it hard?"

"To be stable, shoulders need to have a good relationship between the shoulder blades and rib cage; they have to be 'snug.' My teacher used to say that they need to be in a sort of 'make-out-session.' That means that they are close together, rubbing up against each other, and not playing hard to get." Aurie snorts.

"Hard to get?!" Adam smiles.

"Let me explain. The rib cage plays 'hard to get' when it starts jutting out, especially at the bottom, as the shoulder blades come in towards it. To counter that, we use 3-part breath to ensure that the rib cage is not jutting out and is in fact pressing into the shoulder blades. The shoulder blades can play 'hard to get' as well, so we make sure that our heart is forward, and we are becoming broad in both in the chest and the back. In our 'Practices' workshop we'll talk about how to do this." You sigh a bit, turning the page of your notebook. Your wrist is already hurting a bit from all of the writing that you're doing. You look up, and see Adam preparing to talk more as he chugs on his water bottle one last time."

"Okay guys and girls, hold on, we're almost through this! For now, just know that when you do them skillfully, yoga poses will strengthen the shoulder and help you with mobility. However, in order to maintain healthy alignment in a lot of poses, your shoulders have to already be somewhat strong. So it's important to know which poses require a lot of shoulder strength and which don't. Low plank is a perfect example – if you're not strong enough to keep your shoulders in healthy alignment you not only risk injury, but also build strength unevenly. This uneven buildup of strength will perpetuate a slumping of the shoulders forward, if you already do that."

"The most common misalignment in low plank is to collapse the chest and allow the heads of arm bones forward toward the floor; FHS. When this happens, the shoulder blades poke out instead of lying flat on the back as they should. They are playing hard to get, and you're way out of OSP. Do your best to build your shoulder strength up both inside and outside of your posture practice, and watch your alignment in poses like low plank. Good cues from a teacher help here. When you feel weak, your alignment may suffer even more than usual, so consider modifications or just taking a break." Adam leans back against the white board and looks up at the clock. "Okay, that's stability. Lets jump over to shoulder mobility!"

"It shouldn't be news to hear that our shoulder mobility is often slowly reduced by a habitual repetition of everyday activities. These include driving, sitting in front of a computer, sitting on the couch, maintaining a regular posture of FHS or simply avoiding a full range of motion in the shoulder. I feel like I'm repeating myself here. Like I said, if you don't use it, you lose it. On the bright side, your awareness of your own posture is one of the first steps to increasing shoulder mobility. I think you're already getting that now. Our posture practice is the perfect cure for all of this shoulder trouble. It can help us maintain or increase mobility when it includes poses that require flexion, extension and rotation in the shoulder while still being stable." Adam throws his marker into his bag, and plops down into his chair. It strikes you suddenly that this is the first time you've seen him sit down in his chair since the first day of class.

"We did it guys and gals! We're done! Congratulations, you are now officially ½ of the way through your foundational 'Stretchers' class, and well on your way to becoming a Rhema Yoga yogi or yogini! I hope I didn't go too quickly towards the end here, I know I took less questions, but we were simply way too far behind schedule. Again, feel free to ask me anything online. For now, lets all meditate for a bit, and then we'll end this class. Remember, your midterm is next week, so be sure you study!" As Adam gets up to lower the lights, you grin in spite of the midterm and pack up your bags. The last meditation really hit the spot for you, and after all the data you covered today, a good 5-10 minute session sounds perfect.

CHAPTER 9

THE MIDTERM

Name:_____

Note: Hello student! This is an open book test, so feel to look up any answers you don't know. If you want to learn the most possible from this test, I suggest you try each question without looking the answer up first, and then go back to find the answers later.

There is an answer key to this test at www.rhemayoga.com/stretchermidterm.

Enjoy!

1. What are the 7 Stars?
    a. Something from the book of Genesis
    b. Another word for the 7 locks
    c. Parts of the body
    d. Parts of the core

2. Concentric contraction is a case in which your muscle is shortened and contracted.
    a. True
    b. False
    c. Could be either, depending on the circumstance
    d. None of the above

3. List out the 7 Stars

4. In Rhema Yoga, we are mostly about getting _____ of the lumbar and getting _____ to the thoracic when it comes to twists and bends.

5. The outer spiral is an instance when the muscle rotates around the bone outward, _____ from the front and centerline of the body.

6. What is the main purpose of the muscle locks?
    a. To keep your muscles from getting too relaxed
    b. To rebound your energy and improve alignment in poses
    c. To keep bad energy out of your body
    d. All of the above

7. Why don't we just call it "Rhema Stretching" or "Rhema Postures" or something like that?
    a. Because there is more to yoga than stretching
    b. Because we want to sound cool
    c. Because we couldn't decide between stretching or postures, so we gave up
    d. None of the above

8. Why do knee injuries almost always take longer to heal than muscle injuries?
    a. Because knees are not well made
    b. Because muscles get less blood than knees
    c. Because ligaments, tendons and cartilage get less blood than muscles
    d. B and C

9. What does OSP stand for?
    a. Otter-Snake-Parrot
    b. Optimal Standing Posture
    c. Optimal Standing Pattern
    d. Optimal Stand-Pray

10. Range of motion is the range at which a joint can move both easily and easefully, without needing help from _____.

11. A muscle is made strong and healthy when it is regularly concentrically and eccentrically contracted.
    a. True
    b. False
    c. It depends on whether you are doing yoga or something else
    d. None of the above

12. Foot lock is vital to all of our standing poses because it provides extra _____ to the body.

13. The lumbar curve, like the cervical curve, is _____ in its curve, but unlike the cervical it is the _____ mobile of the three in terms of bending and twisting.

14. What is OSP?
    a. A way to communicate to other people without talking
    b. A posture pattern that is unhealthy and common in the U.S.
    c. A posture pattern that is very healthy and how we were designed to stand, sit and etc.
    d. A posture pattern that is unhealthy, and features a person who leans back too far in the torso. It is the opposite of FHS.

15. What are 5 negative physical affects from FHS that were mentioned in the "Stretchers" class?

16. Other than full ab lock, there are 6 muscle locks. What are they?
    a. Foot lock, knee lock, root lock, ab lock, heart lock, throat lock
    b. Foot lock, knee lock, root lock, ab lock, throat lock, soul lock
    c. Foot lock, root lock, ab lock, heart lock, throat lock, soul lock
    d. None of the above

17. What does FHS stand for?
    a. Fillet-Ham-Sandwich
    b. Forward Hand Syndrome
    c. Forward Head Syndrome
    d. Forward Head Posture

18. What is yoga orphanship?

19. What are the Big 3 for healthy knees?
    a. Ice, Yoga and Ben-Gay
    b. Stability, Structure, Alignment
    c. Structure, Practice, Tension
    d. Stability, Strain, Alignment

20. The quad muscles are a group of _____ muscles that is located _____ the knee.

21. What is the difference between the 7 Stars and the 8 Instances?

22. The quad muscles function to _____ your knee.

23. During your practice, a muscle acting as a mover helps to _____ in all of your postures, and a muscle acting as a stabilizer helps to _____ the movement.

24. What does someone mean when they say the "8 Instances?" What does that mean or describe?

25. Internal rotation is about the movement which rotates the limb, or a part of a limb, _____ towards the _____ of the frontal body."

26. What is FHS?
    a. A posture pattern that most Americans have. It is unhealthy.
    b. A yoga pose that most Americans do, but should not do.
    c. A person who does not like Rhema Yoga. This makes FHS our biggest enemy
    d. A and B

27. The inner spiral is a situation to describe the moment when your muscle _____, toward the front and centerline of the body

28. The core is a major part of our body, and part of the 8 Instances even though it does not describe any particular movement or action.
    a. True
    b. False
    c. None of the Above

29. Eccentric contraction is a time when your muscle is lengthened and contracted.
    a. True
    b. False
    c. None of the Above

30. Sometimes further movement into a pose is inhibited due to bone structure. In this case, it's not muscles stopping you, but a case of bone meeting bone. We call this _____.

31. What are the 4 Legs?
    a.   Something demonic
    b.   Something a dog has
    c.   Meditation, Teaching, Breathing, Postures
    d.   Meditation, Prayer, Breathing, Postures
    e.   Cleansing, Alignment, Posture, Locks

32. When a muscle is stretched to its maximum ability, further movement is inhibited by _____.

33. Stability is dependent on mobility, true or false?
    a.   True
    b.   False
    c.   None of the Above

34. Mobility is the body's ability to partake in all of the various posture movements with ease in both _____ and _____ tissue.

35. What is the "Idea of 4s" in Rhema Yoga?
    a.   Something crazy that Adam made up when he needed sleep
    b.   The idea that we are creating/recreating ourselves in Rhema
    c.   The idea that we are using numbers in all of Rhema Yoga with a special purpose in mind
    d.   The idea that we should do four good things each day

36. List out the 5 Modules.

37. What is yoga sonship?

38. What are the 4 Stretchers?
    a.   Four very good yogis who created Rhema Yoga with Adam
    b.   Inversions, Locks, Alignment, Posture
    c.   Forward bend, backward bend, twist and inversions
    d.   Cleansing, Locks, Alignment, Posture

39. What are the Evil Twins?
    a.   Two scary, life-sized dolls that speak without batteries
    b.   Yoga Orphanship and Incorrect teaching
    c.   Yoga Orphanship and Yoga Sonship

40. List out the 8 Instances

41. What is the difference between the 8 Instances and the 7 Stars?

42. External rotation is a movement at a joint that rotates a limb or some part of a part of your body outward and away from _____.

43. The average twist for a person's lumbar is at least 90%.
    a.   True
    b.   False
    c.   None of the Above

Bonus: Why do the 7 Stars have an "ab core" and the 8 Instances have "core movement?" What is the difference?

ABOUT THE AUTHOR

Originally from New York, Adam is the founder of Rhema Yoga, LLC. He has two Masters degrees, has owned several businesses, and has acted as pastor for several churches in Mainland China (PRC). In his search for truth, Adam has taken on several different worldviews, identities and lifestyles. These include Deadhead/Hippy, Frat Boy, Multinational Consultant, DJ, Catholic, Mormon (LDS), Kung Fu Enthusiast, Evangelical Christian, Business Owner, Air Force Office Training School cadet, Yoga Enthusiast and more.

www.ingramcontent.com/pod-product-compliance
Lightning Source LLC
Chambersburg PA
CBHW060336290526
45793CB00003B/641